10-13-75

THE HOSPITAL/MEDICAL RACKET AND YOU

Books by Rex Dye

The Hospital/Medical Racket and You
Lumber Camp Life in Michigan
Capitalism in a Changing World
A Study of Market Depletion

The Hospital/Medical Racket and You

Rex Dye

An Exposition-Banner Book

Exposition Press   **Hicksville, New York**

Contents

1—Some Highlights of the Problem   7

Thirty to forty percent of doctors making a killing—corrective action should come from within profession—flagrant dishonesty—overloaded "appointment" schedules —hospitals

2—A Case Record of a Specific Hospital Experience   15

A letter from the hospital—the correspondence which brought this letter—further correspondence

3—Observations on Hospital Charges and Costs   28

A comparison of bed charges—Regents hike rates—some incidents of hospital's money hunger—hospital charges passed on to consumer in consumer goods prices—some factors resulting in excessive hospital billing

4—Why Are Hospital/Medical Insurance Rates Skyrocketing?   40

Basic insurance principles not applied—costs which have no place in your hospital bill

5—Hospitalization at Bargain Rates for the Influential and other "Public Relations" Activity   45

Henry Ford Hospital, Detroit, Mich.—St. Joseph Mercy Hospital, Pontiac, Mich.—Providence Hospital, Detroit, Mich.—Sinai Hospital, Detroit, Mich.

6—Keeping the Public in Ignorance   49

A helpless market—monopoly—secrecy

7—The Problem of Producing Doctors   52

   Purpose of medical education—failure of medical educators—the "specialist" and his charges—maintaining doctor
   shortage—China and medical training

8—Political Aspects of the Problem   56
   Correspondence with politicians

9—Bureaucratic Aspects   91

   The futility of bureaucracy

10—Other Economic Aspects   100

   Health care costs and cost of consumer goods

11—Racket Aspects   105

   Dollar motivation—intimidation—bill padding—"or else"
   —conflict of interest

12—Corrective Action   109

   From within the profession—need of public support—
   consumer groups—your local newspaper—needed action

Appendices   115
Recommendations for Further Reading   120
Index   122

1

Some Highlights of the Problem

When Dr. John F. Knowles, former head of Massachusetts General Hospital, now president of the Rockefeller Foundation, said that between 30 and 40 percent of American doctors are making a killing in their practices and that "incredible amounts of unnecessary surgery are going on," the "ethics and discipline" committee of the Massachusetts Medical Society voted to censure him.

The fact that Dr. Knowles was censured for his public statement may indicate why the 60 to 70 percent of doctors who are *not* "making a killing" or doing unnecessary surgery are reluctant to speak out on these abuses and to take action to correct them. Yet it seems to me that this 60 to 70 percent of ethical doctors should take action to correct this exploitation of the helpless and monopolized health market before public and political pressure forces corrective action by the federal government.

There is little evidence that federal bureaucracies would improve the delivery of health services or reduce the skyrocketing costs. Corrective action should come from within the medical profession and men with the courage and understanding of Dr. Knowles should initiate and carry through a housecleaning on a national scale that would rid state and national associations, hospitals and state and federal health departments, of the parasites who have brought medical and health care in the United States to a state of crisis.

The *Detroit Free Press* of September 9, 1973, carried a headline "Chairman of AMA Indicted." Dr. John Kernodle, of Burlington, North Carolina, the AMA chairman, along with five other prominent North Carolinians, was indicted by a federal grand jury on charges of conspiracy and misapplying funds totaling nearly $1.8 million.

7

On April 12, 1974, the *Detroit Free Press* carried a story headed "Hospital Head Quits at U.M." An audit had revealed that Edward Connors, Director of University Hospital, Ann Arbor, Michigan, had doubled-billed approximately $8,000 to the University of Michigan and other organizations in the past three years. University of Michigan president, Robben Fleming, was quoted as having asked counsel to check out whether they had any legal obligation to prosecute. On April 20, 1974 a follow-up story headed "Ex-Hospital Chief to Repay $8,000 He took from U.M." appeared in the *Detroit Free Press*. The regents of the university announced that no criminal charges would be brought. Robben Fleming is said to have stated "The world of health care needs Connor's talents and I am confident he will find a new start for what will yet be recorded as a distinguished career." Fleming did not state whether or not he would give the double-billing director a character reference.

At the same meeting a majority of the regents voted to keep faculty salaries at U.M. secret. Regent Gerald Dunn (D), who introduced the motion for ending salary secrecy said such disclosure was important "in light of the political climate and mistrust of government." The U.M. administration and board of regents have consistently opposed letting the taxpayers know how their money is being spent.

I later learned that the University and Mr. Connors had arrived at a settlement of approximately $15,000 to be paid within three years.

Connors was finally charged by the Michigan attorney general's office with eight counts of obtaining money under false pretenses, seven of which were felonies carrying a maximum penalty of eight years in prison. The assistant attorney general, Michael Materna, said the charges were "out and out easy to prove offenses."

As the audit was said to have revealed $8,000 of double billing and the settlement was for $15,000, the question of the reason for the additional $7,000 in settlement is unanswered.

Judge Ross W. Campbell of the Washtenaw County Circuit Court was to sentence Connors. I wrote Mr. Materna in November of 1974 asking what sentence was given Connors as I saw nothing in the newspapers on this. I have had no response as of December 21, 1974, and am inclined to believe that my request has been ignored. Perhaps political pressure by powerful forces has been applied to avoid further public exposure.

Among those who are "making a killing" in the health market are pathologists and radiologists, some of whom are getting $100,000 a year or more on a "percentage of the take" basis. Dr. James B. Taylor, president of the Southern Illinois Hospital Corporation, Carbondale, Illinois, is reported to have said that a pathologist at his hospital got more than $100,000 a year without ordering, performing, or interpreting more than 90 percent of the laboratory tests!

In 1972, Governor Richard B. Ogilvie of Illinois ordered a review of the qualifications and credentials of all doctors working for the state after it was revealed that 200 patients had died after treatment by a state hospital physician labeled an "impostor." I have seen no follow-up on this story. It would be highly interesting to know the results of this review.

In 1972, University Hospital at Ann Arbor, Michigan, established a "burn center." A "letter to the editor" in the *Detroit Free Press,* November 30, 1972, stated the case of a burn patient hospitalized for eight days received a bill for $5,300, an average of $662 per day.

An analysis of the cost items on this billing by a disinterested cost analyst would be revealing. Such a bill would be a disaster for most families!

On May 18, 1974, the *Detroit Free Press* carried a story on how three doctors, apparently in joint practice, got over $1 million out of the $72 million Medicaid payments in Michigan in 1973. One hundred and ninety-seven doctors collected over $18 million, averaging over $90,000 each. The 11,000 doctors in the state averaged around $5,000 apiece. These fees are of course in addition to their non-Medicaid practice.

The *Detroit Free Press* on July 26, 1974, reported that a senate investigator, David P. Vienna, told Senator Jackson's committee that drug abuse, homosexuality and punitive treatment were widespread at University Center, a psychiatric hospital in Ann Arbor, Michigan, owned by Dr. Arnold H. Kanby and that the hospital had charged the Campus Medical Insurance Program at least $108,000 for services not performed.

On Sunday, August 25, 1974, the *Detroit Free Press* carried a story under the heading "Hospital Murder Probe Continues." The hospital, Petersburg General, at Petersburg Commonwealth, Virginia, suspended LeRoy Hargrave, Jr., a full-time nurses' assistant, after a Pinkerton investigation requested by the hospital. Hargrave, employed in the hospital's coronary care unit was indicted for the murder of Josephine Thomas, a patient. The story stated that a second murder indictment may be sought and as many as ten more bodies may be exhumed in the investigation. Autopsies showed that two patients died from overdoses of Lidocaine during Hargrave's shift from 11 P.M. to 7 A.M.

In Senator William Proxmire's book *Uncle Sam—the Last of the Bigtime Spenders,"** in chapter 9 there is a revealing illustration of how the head of the Food and Drug Administration, Dr. Henry Welch, operated in flagrant conflict of interests as editor of two medical journals in the field of antibiotics. He and his wife also held a half interest in Medical Encyclopedia, Inc., publishers of *Antibiotics Annual.*

While head of the Division of Antibiotics for seven years, Welch received over $287,000 from his publishing interests in the drug industry. He was during this period a full-time government employee, a "public servant" collecting a substantial salary from taxpayers while functioning in the interests of the "health industry"!

Welch avoided an appearance before the Kefauver Investigating Committee, no prosecution was undertaken and he was allowed to quietly resign with "a tap on the wrist," says Proxmire.

If hospital/medical combines can place their representatives in such crucial spots as the Food and Drug Administration, and if caught get them out of trouble with "a tap on the wrist" what protection has the public?

It is possible, yet not probable, that the federal government may act to clean house at the F.D.A. The *Detroit Free Press* ran a news item August 25, 1974, headed "F.D.A. Policies Probed by U.S.," stating that the government would conduct a review of charges by eleven F.D.A. scientists and three outside advisors of drug industry favoritism,

---

*William Proxmire, *Uncle Sam—The Last of the Bigtime Spenders* (New York: Simon & Schuster, 1972).

improper practices and harassment, before a joint hearing of two senate subcommittees.

Casper W. Weinberger, secretary of the Department of Health, Education and Welfare, said a panel of six "experts" would be named to examine the complaints and report within six months. Such an investigation should be completed in thirty days by a competent team, but bureaucrats put decisions as far into the future as possible and action on the report to be made six months in the future may be subject to drug industry influence and control.

The *Washtenaw News Review,* Ann Arbor, Michigan, carried a story headlined "Medicaid Abuse Unchecked." It stated that in the last 18 months seven Michigan physicians had been prosecuted by the federal government for Medicare fraud but that the state was not interested in "that route" on Medicaid fraud.

Of the seven prosecuted by the federal government for Medicare fraud only one was listed as a high pay provider under Medicare, Dr. James D. Payne of Bay City, Michigan, who got away with $127,663 under the Michigan Medicare program. He agreed to repay the state $35,000 of this bonanza! The article did not state how much additional money he got from his Medicare fraud for which he is awaiting sentence by the federal district court.

On August 28, 1974 in "Letters to the Editor," *Detroit Free Press,* a grandparent told of a four-year-old grandson taken to Children's Hospital, Detroit, with a cut finger. After soaking the finger and applying a bandage, no stitches, they got a bill for forty dollars! The money hunger of hospitals apparently knows no limits!

In addition to the fact that costs of health services are exorbitant there is the fact that the quality of these services is often inferior.

An Oakland County Michigan, circuit judge, Frederick C. Ziem, issued a restraining order against Dr. Jesse Ketchum to stop practicing in Michigan, April 30, 1974. Ketchum had already been convicted of criminally negligent homicide by a New York court. An eleven-page complaint was filed by Oakland County prosecutor, L. Brooks Peterson. A ten-year history of malpractice and criminal action against Ketchum showed that he had been charged three times in Michigan for illegal abortions, convicted for federal income tax evasion, and leaving a needle in a thirteen-year-old patient's throat which was discovered two years later by another doctor.

Where were the federal, state and local health authorities; the national, state and local medical associations; the members of the medical profession, during this ten-year period? Why didn't ethical doctors act to rid the profession of such a "doctor"?

This may be due in part to the fact that the doctor or the hospital is more interested in your pocketbook than in your health. When you make an appointment with a doctor for a specific time and are kept waiting for a half hour or more, I feel that the doctor may be one of those out to "make a killing." Your "appointment" simply gives you the privilege of waiting until he processes preceding "appointments" and can spare you a few minutes of his time. His mind and interest may well be on the patients following you and he cannot give you enough time or attention for proper professional diagnosis of your trouble.

No other professional man would even consider making "appointments" without regard for the time of the client. If he did, he would soon be out of business! Doctors who overload their appointment schedules and do not even extend the courtesy of telling the patient of the delay have an arrogant disregard for the value of your time.

This practice of overloading appointment schedules can also be lucrative to the doctor. The doctor gives the patient a prescription and tells the patient to see him again in x number of days which assures more office visits and helps maintain the overloaded and highly profitable appointment schedule. If your case becomes serious and time-consuming he can always send you to a hospital. This helps maintain the highly profitable "production line" office traffic and he can still collect for his calls at the hospital or nursing home where he can spend a few minutes with each of his patients there.

But when you or one of your loved ones enters a hospital, the problem of health care becomes even more serious and costly. Hospital charges are exorbitant and often have no relation to actual, real costs and the amounts charged to patients. This aspect will be dealt with more fully later.

You have little or no choice when it comes to health. You are a "buyer" in a market which is beyond your range of knowledge. You choose a doctor on faith or on someone else's reference. From then on you are in his hands and at his mercy. If he sends you to a hospital, he selects the hospital. There is no competitive market and no price control. In any event, you are in no position to bargain. Cost is no objective in times of severe illness—and those who are out to "make a killing" are fully aware of this fact and profit by it.

The callous treatment of patients in many hospitals can become a horror story. In a letter to Ann Landers appearing in the *Detroit Free Press,* December 21, 1971, the writer of the letter stated that her father-in-law was hospitalized in a room with two other men one of whom died at 1:15 P.M. The corpse was left in the room until 8:30 P.M. Ann Landers in her response stated "according to the physicians with whom I discussed this macabre incident, where hospitals are concerned these days, ANYTHING is possible—and it is becoming more so every year." I would assume that Ann Landers has confidential access to fully qualified physicians and that the foregoing statement would never have been made and printed without good authority.

Hospitals appear to be controlled by an academic "elite" whose primary motivations seem to revolve around a desire for professional prestige involving exotic operations such as heart transplants and brain surgery, securing complex, sophisticated and costly hospital equipment whether or not it is needed or duplicates already existing equipment in the area, adequate to meet all real area needs. In addition to this, we have the motivation of greed and status based on financial incentives. Hospitals are notoriously money conscious, and money hungry, even the "nonprofit" organizations. And as hospital services are sold to an unprotected, uninformed, noncompetitive and captive market by hospitals, opportunity for the exploitation of that market is virtually unlimited.

University Hospital at Ann Arbor, Michigan, a facility of the university, issued a bulletin "Highlights of Balance Sheet" as of June 30, 1970, which showed they had cash "invested" with the University of Michigan totaling $1,935,000. Now this hospital is a tax free, "nonprofit" activity of the university operating under "constitutional autonomy" which permits a high degree of secrecy as to salaries and other expenditures. The $1,935,000 "invested" could only result from an excess of income over costs, in other words, in actuality a "profit," even though this is a nonprofit state facility. I have been unable to secure any information as to why this profit was not used to reduce charges to patients, how this profit was invested with the university, what returns the hospital received on this investment or if the investment was ever liquidated.

The reluctance of University of Michigan management to let the public know about their financial operations was illustrated by a story in the *Detroit Free Press* on December 11, 1974, headlined "Hoarding of Funds" which stated that the auditor general's office of the state of Michigan charged that the University had $44.3 million in "special accounts" apart from its general operating fund. Invested at the prime rate of around 10 percent, this would produce a revenue of over $4 million annually, but the taxpayers of Michigan are apparently not to be let in on this even though tuition rates are hiked and demands for funds from university officials soar. Full investigation of salaries, expense accounts and other financial "operations" here and at the University Hospital appear to be long overdue.

Taxpayers are not supposed to ask where their money goes and if they are so persistent in the face of academic arrogance as to ask for such information it is refused them. If the taxpayer tries to get information from state agencies or political figures he will find the response, if any, tactfully ducks the issue, with, however, exceptions from those few who really function in the public interest. More detailed light on this question will appear later in this volume.

2

A Case Record of a Specific Hospital Experience

Until June 12, 1970, I had had little experience with hospitals from the standpoint of a user of hospital services. My wife had for several months been afflicted with an illness having the symptoms of rheumatoid arthritis. University Hospital at Ann Arbor, Michigan, was reported by a local arthritis association to have special facilities in this area, and after discussion with our family physician we decided to hospitalize her in this hospital for diagnosis and treatment. She was admitted on June 12, 1970, and after three weeks was discharged on July 3, 1970, with a diagnosis of terminal cancer.

I was told by three different doctors that, with the equipment and facilities here, the diagnosis could have been made in half the time—and they were emphatic in their refusal to have their names used in any way. The service was poor and I became shockingly aware of the inefficiency and inadequacy of patient care in hospitals.

I wrote University Hospital outlining my observations and received this letter in response:

UNIVERSITY HOSPITAL
September 22, 1970

Mr. Rex Dye
525 Harper Avenue
Detroit, Michigan 48202

Dear Mr. Dye:
Your letter outlining some of your observations at our hospital was carefully reviewed, with several areas of our hospital organization, which you

15

outlined. Mr. Connors who has recently been appointed the new Director of University Hospital, is making special note of the comments which you related in your letter. We are presently in the re-organization process of all aspects of the hospital organization, from top to bottom in this institution, to correct the situations which you so ably pointed out.

Personnel control procedures, hospital charges, the methods of delivery of services, the use of automated equipment and new changes in supervision are now in process to place the Institution on a new course.

The number of matters which you brought to our attention from the viewpoint of a user of hospital services has *been one of the most constructive letters which could have been received by management.* We appreciate your concern and to take the time to detail your reactions, for it will be a factual basis on which our present re-organizing efforts can be based.

Sincerely yours,

John J. Zugich
Associate Director

JJZ:ac

The letter which brought this response was in the form of a memo and follows:

Memo to: UNIVERSITY HOSPITAL
Subject: Costs of Hospitalization—University Hospital, Ann Arbor, Mich.

Based on my observations during the period covered by the attached copy of billing for hospitalization of my wife, it is my belief that charges for hospital services are from two to three times what a fair charge based on realistic costs under efficient operation should be.

Bed Charges: $55 per day (ward). This includes bed, meals, and services of attendants on signal button.

Vastly superior service including meals, room with two beds, privacy, far better attention to patient is available at Beverly Manor Convalescence Centers (operating very successfully under private enterprise *for profit*) at $17 per day.

Based on 1,000 beds at $55 per day, University Hospital has a potential revenue of $20,075 *per bed* per year. One thousand beds equals $20,075,000 per year. This charge is over three times that of the charge made for far better services at the center above mentioned.

Excessive Bed Time: Patient was under the attention of a "team" of young doctors serving an apprenticeship to gain experience prior to entering private practice. The result of this system is an excessive number of lab

tests with days of delay in securing lab findings and action on them resulting in greatly increased bed time (at $55 per day!) and excessive lab
charges.

In my opinion, an experienced diagnostician should be able to determine
probable causes of the condition and by a prompt series of eliminating tests
and examination isolate the cause in less than half the time and lab tests
taken in this case (21 days).

Excessive Laboratory Charges: I am informed by reliable authority that
the laboratory tests used charged out to the patient at from $5 to $15 per test
can, with equipment available today, be produced and sold at a profit above
real cost for a fraction of the amounts charged.

Charges other than bed charge such as laboratory fees, X-rays, "physical
therapy" and medicine averaged $43 per day. This charge (based on 1,000
beds) comes to a total of $43,000 per day or potential charges other than
bed time of $15,695,000 annually. Extensive surgery, etc., would substantially
increase this figure.

Physical Therapy: The subject billing includes $66 in charges for "physi-
cal therapy" at $8 to $10 per visit (a few minutes of exercise of right arm
and left leg) *which, in this case, due to weakening of bone structure caused
by nature of the disease, might be actually detrimental.* (Time of the thera-
pist is apparently charged out at $25 or more per hour!)

Violation of Privacy: During stay here, a group of individuals, apparently
on a guided tour of the establishment, stopped at the bed of my wife while
the conductor of the tour recited information to the group apparently about
her case, without the common courtesy of introduction or asking permission—as though we were specimens on exhibit for the public view! The
fact that such an intrusion might frighten and worry the helpless and
desperately sick patient apparently did not occur to the group. I deeply
resented this callous treatment but due to the condition of my wife said
nothing.

Apparent Causes of Delay and Excessive Costs:

1. Lack of supervision and organization control

   (A) Three times while I was present service button at bed was
       pressed with no response within a reasonable time. I walked
       to desk where lights showed. Girl at desk was busy chatting
       over phone paying no attention to lights. Proper supervision
       would quickly bring this negligence to an end.

   (B) I went to office one afternoon to take care of some paperwork.
       I was told the two women who handled this would be back
       later. No one knew when! Over an hour later they came in,
       in a big hurry, with parcels—apparently having been shopping
       during work hours. Proper supervision would not permit such
       laxity.

   (C) Requests to floor personnel to talk with any of the doctors brought a response that they did not know where they were or when they would be available. Proper supervision would schedule their time and have information available—and save hours of wasted time and strain.

(D) Lab tests, "physical therapy" etc., were carried out without consultation or information to patient—who is left in doubt and uncertainty throughout. Proper supervision would schedule indicated tests to find rapidly by elimination the cause of malady—and the work of laboratory technicians would be brought under effective controls to assure processing efficiently without wasted time or excessive costs to patient.

It is my opinion that effective personnel control procedures could enable this hospital to process twice the number of patients annually, particularly in view of the laboratory and technical equipment this organization has at its disposal with no increase in payroll costs and with definite improvement in the service rendered. This would greatly reduce cost of hospital insurance coverage. [With reference to the author's experience and authority to make this statement see Appendix 2-3.]

It appears that this organization is so loose and lacking in effective controls and the upper management so far removed from the actualities of its operation, that patients become simply numbers and any regard for or understanding of human feeling is lost as well as effective control of the man-hours represented by its payroll.

I wrote Mr. Connors, director of the hospital, regarding the letter from Mr. Zugich:

Dear Mr. Connors:
In response to my letter and memo to you of September 3, 1970, I received a letter from your Mr. John J. Zugich, September 22, acknowledging the validity of my statements as to excessive charges and nature of the services received. Mr. Zugich referred to this communication as "one of the most constructive which could have been received by management." In my letter to you, I enclosed a check for $1,310.81 balance in full of a bill totaling $1,869.81, an amount I believe to be at least three times what reasonable billing based on realistic costs and proper service should have been.

A week later, I received from your financial offices a billing for this balance with a handwritten "dunning" note thereon to the effect that I was delinquent on my obligation in spite of the fact that I paid the amount *in full* 60 days in advance of my commitment at time of admission. This is indicative first, of the laxity and time lapse on handling work and records and second, of the callous attitude hospital personnel have toward patients and their problems.

The hospital had no ethical reluctance to accept this money in spite of the fact that, in my opinion, services and the manner in which they were rendered could not justify such acceptance. If I were to handle problems of my own clients in such an unprofessional manner, with so little regard for their interests and bill them with so little regard for reasonable costs, I would be out of business in 90 days!

Mr. Zugich stated that you are undertaking a reorganization from "top to bottom" and I wish you every success in this program for the problems you face to accomplish this are appalling!

At the "top" you have the medical profession so isolated from the realities of sound administration and so involved in their own pet interests and specialties that the *public interest* involved in meeting the needs of patients in a 1,000 bed hospital and getting the *maximum performance* from these facilities in terms of time and money is, perhaps, beyond their comprehension.

At the "bottom" you have several thousand people probably grown accustomed to lax supervision, lack of direction, control and real job training.

And between the "top" and the "bottom" you have a supervisory structure apparently with no clear lines of authority or responsibility and with no control system to measure performance.

I hope that you will be able to secure the full support of those in high enough places to carry out your program of effective reorganization.

I am sincerely,
Rex Dye

RD:ad

I received in response the following typical political letter of assurance, a letter which says nothing, "appreciates comments," and totally ignores the problem:

Dear Mr. Dye:
I appreciate the comments in your letter of November 12. Rest assured that we will do everything we can to insure that University Hospital serves as an effective organization for the citizens of Michigan.

Sincerely,
Edward J. Connors

EJC:lj

The above letter with its broad generalization as to "service to citizens" is obviously an evasion of the issues outlined in my letter and is indicative of the attitude of hospital administration toward the public.

Seven months after my wife died I received a questionnaire from the hospital asking how she was progressing, in spite of the fact that their records would show that this was a terminal case with only weeks to live after discharge. I replied as follows:

Dear Mr. Connors:
I would appreciate your asking Wanda Mildrum to discontinue sending me any further questionnaires such as those enclosed. They only serve to remind me of a very painful experience and her records should show, in this case, how inappropriate and thoughtless such communications are.

I believe this is another illustration of the need for thorough house-cleaning at the hospital, the callous approach to patient's problems and needless costs charged against bed time already about three times what more space and better accommodations provided by private enterprise operating for profit is supplying.

Sincerely,
Rex Dye

Mr. Zugich replied for Mr. Connors as follows:

Dear Mr. Dye:
We are extremely sorry to hear about the questionnaire which you called our attention to. This questionnaire had been designed by our medical staff members as part of our Cancer Registry. The purpose is to maintain research and statistical studies on patients who have had a diagnosis of this important condition and to determine the results of treatment, recurrence, or nonrecurrence. The University Hospital has been cited as having one of the finest follow-up programs in the country, in this area which is used by the American Cancer Society and the American College of Surgeons, in evaluating cancer treatment programs, for the benefit of all future patients nationally. Our inquiries are made annually of 12,000 former patients, covering a period of many years. That is the purpose of the questionnaire and Registry.

This does not, however, obviate the questions which you raised about the appropriateness of the questionnaire form. In view of your letter we shall work with the committee of physicians responsible for the Cancer Registry and follow-up to completely revise the inquiry and still obtain the desirable information to help combat and resolve eventually the treatment of this disease, for the eventual benefit of all. You may rest assured that these changes will be made.

Progress is being made in our re-organization, with many changes taking place in both supervisory personnel methods and attitudes. We trust that these changes for a large organization would meet in a large measure some of the points which you had brought to our attention in your previous correspondence.

Sincerely yours,
John J. Zugich
Associate Director

JJZ:ac

As a specialist in varied research projects involving questionnaires, I considered this questionnaire crude and amateurish. More important, however, is the fact that this "research" activity apparently had no contact with the records which showed this case to be terminal! Statistics based on such unreliable record studies may keep high-salaried members of a "research" staff on the payroll but can be of little help in solving the problems of cancer treatment.

I wrote Mr. Zugich as follows:

Dear Mr. Zugich:

I greatly appreciate your letter of April 1st and am glad to hear that you are making progress in your reorganization plans.

You outline the research activities of your Cancer Registry. In this regard, it seems to me that, were the symptoms of known, comparable cases properly classified and promptly available, then when a case such as that of my wife entered the hospital and symptoms were checked against prior case experience where same symptoms were reported, diagnosis could be made in less than half the time taken in this case.

I am visualizing an automated system of case records carrying punch cards covering varied symptom pattern breakdowns and probable diagnoses. When a case is received, symptoms would be punched on a card, then the card run through the comparison matching unit and *probable* diagnosis would bring final diagnosis quickly—and save many days of costly bed time, eliminate much needless laboratory expense as well as costly "physical therapy" where, as in the case of my wife, it could not possibly serve any desirable purpose.

This would serve not only to cut hospitalization costs to patient and help reduce medical/hospital insurance costs but also, in cases of terminal illness, make it possible for patients to spend more of their final hours on earth in a much more desirable environment and with those they are soon to leave.

Of course, such a system would completely change the system of intern "medical teams." In the case of my wife, at least three different members of such a "team" did the same series of diagnostical questions. (I assume the other members of the "team" did the same in order to gain experience!)

One such series of questions with data transferred to a punch card would be enough.

Many needless laboratory tests, x-rays, etc., would be eliminated as well as lengthy discussions, etc., by members of the student team. Of course, these young doctors would not get the same postgraduate educational experience as they do under the system in effect in 1970—but I do not believe a patient in the hospital should be used to this extent as a subject through which budding doctors can gain experience.

On the other hand, these young men might gain much more knowledge through study of valid case record data and the ultimate diagnoses, as above noted.

I am,

Sincerely,
Rex Dye

I received no response to this communication.

Lou Graff of the University Hospital publicity staff sent me a copy of Edward T. Hall's *The Silent Language,** a very interesting study of the semantics of actions as contrasted with words. I responded with the following letter applying Hall's theories to the hospital/medical culture as it exists at University Hospital.

Lou:
I found *The Silent Language* by Edward T. Hall interesting. Have gone through it once and am reviewing it for essentials of theory.

An analysis of the hospital/medical subculture, based on Hall's thinking would be provocative.

He states: "What people do is more important than what 'they say.' " (Of course, "saying" is a form of "doing" and subject to analysis as an *act*.)

Take University Hospital with some 3,000 employees with regard to two of Hall's "PMS."‡

    (A) "Interaction": speech, specialized vocabulary, largely in a virtually dead language, not understood by laymen and isolating the hospital/medical culture from patient/public culture so that communication between the two cultures is difficult or impossible.

---

*Edward T. Hall, *The Silent Language* (New York: Doubleday & Company, Inc., 1959).

‡"Primary Message Systems."

(B) "Association": 3,000 individuals in this hospital organization with an established "pecking" order, varying degrees of hostility to authority such as you mentioned over the phone, an "elite" group at the top unable to "communicate" with the mass group at bottom, and the impersonal carrying out of established routines without real interest or involvement in the patient as such. (Examples will follow.)

The end result is that the patient becomes a "case"—an anonymous object viewed with the lack of emotional awareness applied to a piece of steel on an automotive production line. The personal dissatisfactions of personnel, personal ambitions of interns looking forward to profitable private practice, insecurities and conflicting interests of supervisory personnel are all reflected in what is "done" rather than "said."

The stimuli received by the nervous systems of personnel as a bloc apparently are discharged into flexor reaction channels more often than extensor with the result that real interest in patient problems and welfare are minimized.

Examples of communication on the level of "what is done rather than said" will, in my experience, include:

(1) Group of several individuals were conducted to my wife's bed— some explanation of case given by leader of group. It probably did not occur to any of this group that their presence could worry and disturb my wife or that a right of privacy was being violated. What was "done" or "communicated" was that they were far more interested in showing hospital facilities, types of cases, etc., than in patient well-being.

(2) During my presence three (3) different interns asked virtually the same series of diagnostic questions of my wife. I have no doubt that the other three members of the team did likewise. It probably did not occur to any of these young men that they were subjecting the patient to needless strain and worry. What was "done" "communicated" a desire for experience for subsequent use in their future private practice rather than welfare of patient as one such interview, properly recorded, would produce all information that could be had orally.

(3) (a) Three different times during my presence no response resulted from use of push button at bed even after extended waiting period. Each time I found that the girl at central station was engaged in telephone conversation paying no attention to lights.

(b) I went to the office regarding some paperwork that was needed. The two women who handled this were out and no one knew when they would be back. I returned later and after a considerable wait both returned, with packages, apparently having been shopping during working hours.

The two incidents above "communicate" a lack of concern for the best interests of both hospital and patient and support the thought outlined under (B) "Association" above.

(4) My wife entered the hospital 6/12/70 and was discharged 7/3/70 with diagnosis terminal cancer.

Yet she was given "physical therapy" 6/19, 6/24 and 6/25; 6/29, 6/30, 7/1 and 7/2. Due to the nature of the disease and its effect on bone structure, this physical movement of limbs could have no beneficial effect and may have been harmful, particularly in the last week before discharge. What was "communicated" here supports comment in (B) "Association" above.

(5) I told one of the young doctors on the "team" I would like a copy of the final report on this case. He told me he did not believe I could get one and that *I would need a dictionary to read it!* This amused me! What he "communicated" was that I was not competent to use reference works, should not seek knowledge in this field and that "communication" was impossible. This supports remarks in (A) "Interaction" above.

(6) I received a final bill from the hospital with a handwritten notation "dun" on its face "pay at once." This bill was received 9/8/70. The account had been paid in full 9/2/70, a week before the dunning notice was sent. Needless to say the "communication" conveyed was not calculated to improve public relations for the hospital.

(7) In March of 1971, I received a questionnaire from the hospital addressed to my wife, who died in August of 1970. Hospital records must have shown this to be a terminal case with death a matter of weeks, yet the established "culture" routine carried on, indicating not only a lack of communication between departments, as does (6) above, but also a complete lack of sympathy for, or understanding of, the problems faced by survivors, reflecting "hospital culture" mental states outlined in (B) "Association" above.

(8) "Association" (B) above, is further exemplified by the established "culture" routine which results in excessive "bed time," delay in "diagnosis time" and excessive charges to patient. Hall's comment on the "language of time" is illuminating when applied to the "hospital culture." (3) (a) and (b) above illustrate two facets of "time" language I found here. *My* "time" and "time" of patient were of no consequence in spite of the very real urgency from our frame of reference. "Time" of employee applied to our interests had an entirely different value as did "time" of employee paid for by the hospital.

In the foregoing, I have reviewed this general situation largely from the frame of reference outlined in the theories developed by Hall in the work you so kindly sent me.

One might go further with a study based on Korzybski's* theories of general semantics—the "communication" resulting from "semantic reactions on the cortical as well as thalamic levels—the "multi-ordinal" nature of "meaning" whether verbal or non-verbal—"conditional" reactions resulting from environmental and job conditioning—but bringing order out of such chaos is a monumental undertaking!

How are you going to "communicate" to employees the fact that their lack of feeling for, or real interest in, the welfare of a patient causes suffering and heartache?

How are you going to "communicate" to young interns that the welfare of patients before them is of far more importance than their possible future careers as doctors?

How are you going to "communicate" to your upper professional levels the fact that the primary immediate purpose of a hospital is: give the best possible kind, considerate, compassionate and expeditious care at lowest possible cost to those so unfortunate as to require hospital care?

And, with regard to *costs,* please refer to the data enclosed. Why should patients, forced to resort to hospital care under severe physical and emotional pressure, be forced to pay for goods and services they do not receive such as research costs, student training, etc., etc.? Why should insurance rates be based on such costs?

Surely research and student training are needed—but should be paid for by the public at large through national and state funding for these activities are "futures" for *general* good and can have little benefit for the immediate patient.

If such charges are to be passed on to patients they should be in the open as specific items on billing, not as hidden costs concealed from the patient as general charges.

I enjoyed our phone conversation and thanks for Hall's book which I am going through again with the view of relating his thought to Korzybski's analyses.

Sincerely,
Rex Dye

Mr. Graff replied:

Dear Mr. Dye,
I genuinely appreciated your letter of October 18, particularly for your very astute critique of the Hall book.

---

*Alfred Korzybski, *Science and Sanity,* 4th ed. (Connecticut: International Non-Aristotelian Library Publishing Co., 1958).

Much of the delay in my response is due to a combination of personal illness, and unyielding pressure of urgent assignments, and an effort to get you the answers to the specific questions in your letter.

I'm not sure that I can satisfy you even now. However, the following information comes from Mr. E. C. Laetz, Associate Director for the Hospital in charge of financial affairs. He provided me with the following information:

"A statement of account dated 8/27/70 was sent to Mr. Rex Dye in the amount of $1,319.81. Mr. Dye states that he received this notice on September 8, 1970. It is difficult to determine at this late date why it took so long for this notice to be received by Mr. Dye.

"Mr. Dye stated that he paid this account in full on September 2, 1970, yet his letter of transmittal, dated September 3, undoubtedly did not reach the hospital until Friday, September 4, 1970. This was the Friday just before Labor Day. Undoubtedly, the receipt of this money was not officially noted until September 8, 1970. Attached is a photocopy of the notice sent and his notation in a return of that notice.

"Mrs. Dye was hospitalized on 6 West where the room charge at that time was $45 per day. On July 1 she was moved into a semi-private room where the rate was $55 a day. She died on July 3. The increase from $45 to $55 can be explained by the fact that room rates were increased as of July 1."

I also obtained from Mr. Laetz a copy of the balance sheet of University Hospital, which you are welcome to have. I am really not equipped to answer any questions on the balance sheet myself, so I suggest if you have any questions, that you feel free to call or write Mr. Laetz directly.

I would like to meet you for lunch sometime when I am in Detroit so that I might get some suggestions from you both because of your personal experiences and because of your professional background in the media as to what you think might be done specifically out of my office to improve our patient and public relations efforts.

Yours truly,
Louis Graff, Director
Health Sciences Relations

In my response to Mr. Graff's preceding letter in paragraph two I called attention to two errors of fact and in paragraph four asked a question which has not yet been answered—why did University Hospital, a nonprofit, nontaxpaying facility charge three times as much for beds as a taxpaying enterprise operating for profit? This question will be more fully developed in the next chapter. My letter to Mr. Graff follows.

Dear Lou:

Your thoughtful letter of November 15th was welcome and your interest in this overall hospital/medical situation is appreciated.

In paragraph six of your letter quoting Mr. Laetz, there appears to be two errors. (1) Mrs. Dye was not moved to a semi-private room to my knowledge and billing item of 6/30/70 shows "$45 Ward WO 6630, 19 days"—item of 7/2/70 $55 Ward in WO 6630, 2 days" (no billing of semi-private room). (2) She did not *die* on July 3rd but was discharged. (Died August 14th, at Beverly Manor.) I was told by one of the interns that *ward rate* was increased to $55 per day as of July 1st.

All of this is, however, more or less beside the point, as the real issue is, I believe, concerned with the costs, organization and efficiency of hospitals in general and the attitudes, objectives and motivations of hospital personnel (which establish and control their "silent language" and which has brought to hospital/medical "culture" under severe criticism nationally).

I would like to see an analysis of costs used to determine bed charges as it is impossible for me to understand why, if an institution such as Beverly Manor Convalescent Centers operating around 4,000 beds in widely varied geographical areas, can provide the type of service they do for $17 per day at a profit and pay taxes. (See accompanying data.) Why can not hospitals at least sell bed time on a comparable basis?

I'll be glad to get together with you for lunch any time you're in town. Just phone me any morning, as I keep my time fairly open.

It is my feeling that the question of improving public/patient relations is at this time, primarily an internal one with hospitals, largely as outlined in my letter of October 18th. Two fundamental problems seem to exist; (1) "humanizing" service; (2) substantially reducing cost. I have talked to many people who have had experiences with hospitals during the past year and these two reactions seem universal.

Sincerely,
Rex Dye

3

Observations on Hospital Charges and Costs

After my wife was discharged from University Hospital she entered the Beverly Manor Convalescent Center within a mile of our home. She occupied a tastefully arranged two-bed room with one other patient. The room was spacious with closets for clothes and a connected bath. Meals were far better than those at the hospital. When the call button was used it was answered promptly by pleasant, efficient personnel with real interest in the comfort of the patient. The charge for this bed and service was $17 per day, *less* than one-third the charge made by the hospital, in spite of the fact that this convalescent home was operated for profit and paid taxes while University Hospital was a "non-profit" state facility paying no taxes. One should keep clearly in mind that the services provided were identical in kind, though far different in quality. The patient is put in the position of an automobile buyer forced to pay $9,000 for a car that could be bought elsewhere for $3,000.

Medical and laboratory charges were separate items in addition to the charge for beds in both cases.

A comparison of services and charges follows:

Beverly Manor   *University Hospital*

SPACE

(1) *Area per bed*—(see diagram) approximately 5 times the area per bed provided by University Hospital plus bath and wardrobes.

(1) *Area per bed*—(see diagram) bed surrounded by canvas-pull curtain—barely room for visitor chair—no bath—no wardrobe.

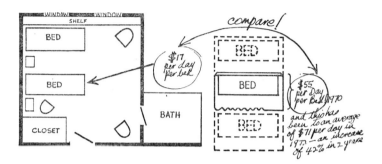

Beverly Manor	*University Hospital*

(2) *Maintenance*—At equal cost per sq. ft., cost per bed much higher here.

(2) *Maintenance*—Minimum cost per bed due to restricted area per bed.

(3) *Capital Investment*—Much higher cost per bed.

(3) *Capital Investment*—As a state-owned facility, cost borne by taxpayers. Even if privately operated, investment should have been amortized rapidly based on charges made.

(4) *Heat and Light*—At equal cost per sq. ft. of bed space would be much higher here.

(5) *Insurance*

(6) *Real Estate, personal property and income taxes*—A private enterprise paying substantial taxes to federal and state governments.

(6) Does University Hospital as a state-owned institution pay any of these taxes? (No)

MEALS

Excellent

Fair—Volume buying and processing should make costs lower than at Beverly Manor.

Beverly Manor	*University Hospital*

HOUSEKEEPING AND LAUNDRY

Much neater, cleaner and more attractive.	Volume processing should make this cost lower than at Beverly Manor.

BED SERVICE
(Call Button)

Prompt, pleasant and efficient response by competent personnel.	Delayed response, not as high-type personnel.

CHARGES

$17 per day	$55 per day

Excess charged by University Hospital—$38 per day.

Based on 1,000 beds at University Hospital this amounts to an excess charge of $38,000 per day.

This does not take into account the fact that Beverly Manor is operated by private enterprise *for profit, with costs far greater than those that could be fairly charged against bed space at University Hospital.*

Were an institution such as Beverly Manor to provide bed space such as that at University Hospital such facilities could probably be provided at a profit at a cost to the patient not in excess of $10 per day as against the $55 per day charged by University Hospital.

Keep in mind that all you get for $55 per day at this hospital is the privilege of using a bed as above noted. All other services such as medical care, operating rooms, x-rays, laboratory services, "physical therapy," medicine, etc., are *extra* and billed at highest rates.

University Hospital provides nothing in the way of bed space or *service* for $55 per day not available in the convalescent home cited at a charge of $17 per day.

University Hospital is charging approximately $20,000,000.00 a year for services that could be obtained elsewhere at a much higher level of service in a much better environment for approximately $6,000,000.00 a year

This is very important. Where does the extra $38,000 per day go? Is this hidden cost the charge levied against patients and insuring companies to pay for training of medical students, research regarding which no information as to objectives, accomplishment, or costs appears to be available, and excessive salaries to a privileged group?

Laboratory service was provided by a commercial laboratory fifteen miles from the convalescent home. This laboratory had transportation costs, paid taxes and operated for profit, yet charges were approximately 20 percent lower than at the hospital with laboratories in their own building, paying no taxes and *not* operating for profit.

In an effort to secure information on figures used to establish the bed charge of $55 per day I wrote the hospital as follows:

Mr. Edward J. Connors, Director
University Hospital
Ann Arbor, Michigan

Dear Mr. Connors:
Please send me operating figures and balance sheet on 1970 operations of University Hospital and costs used in determining ward bed charge of $55 per day.

Also, what are the salary scales of top hospital personnel, pathologists, etc.?

Thanking you, I am,

Sincerely,
Rex Dye

No response was received in answer to this letter. Such data was a deep, dark secret!

In the *Washtenaw News Review* of July 27, 1972, under the headline "Regents Hike Rates for U Hospital Rooms," it was revealed that the University of Michigan Regents had approved, effective September 1, 1972, increases in daily bed charges from $64 to $73 in large wards and $65 to $70 in small wards. In 1970 these accommodations were $55 per day.

Two-bed private rooms, similar to the rooms at the convalescent home previously cited at $17 per day in 1970, were increased from $66 to $75 daily, an increase of 60 percent in less than two years.

In justifying these increases, the hospital director, Edward J. Connors, was quoted as saying "The new rates are required because of increase in payroll expenses as well as increases in the cost of supplies, equipment, utilities and other commodity costs."

The fact is that in the all items category statistics of the U.S. Department of Labor which include wages, salaries, equipment, utilities and other commodities show that, while all items went from slightly over 100 on the index in 1960 to slightly under 140 in 1970, hospital charges skyrocketed from under 120 on the index to over 280. This still-continuing increase in hospital charges appears to have no causal relationship to general inflation causes and suggests that the exorbitant increase in hospital services is caused by other factors than those resulting in the inflation of charges in all other categories. Among such causes might be found a degree of inefficiency which would be tolerated in no other economic area, exploitation of a captive and helpless market and a defacto covert monopoly functioning with no controls over its activities.

The Washtenaw News Review reported in their July 3, 1974 issue that the University of Michigan Regents had approved an overall rate increase for all hospital service at University Hospital averaging 9 per cent above their previously exorbitant rates. It seems obvious that regents go along with whatever the hospital suggests with no investigation of real costs versus charges made or desired and with little regard for the public interest in a state facility supported by taxpayers' money.

In an attempt to make a clarification of the procedures followed by the regents in permitting this rate increase, I sent the following memo to each of the regents.

Memo to: Regents, University of Michigan
Subject: Rates, University Hospital

In allowing rate increases at University Hospital, Ann Arbor, from $50 per day in 1970 to $71 per day in 1972, an increase of 41 percent in less than two years, were these questions asked of, and answered by, the hospital administration?

(1) Why were bed charges in 1970 $55 per day in wards when far

better bed accommodations were available in semi-private (2 bed) rooms for $17 per day? (Supporting data on request.)

(2) Was the extra $38 per day charge made to support student training and "research"? And, if so, *is this a legitimate and fair expense to be charged to patients?*

(3) Trend Statement, University Hospital 1970 showed $1,935,000 "invested" with University of Michigan. *Why was this "profit" not used to reduce charges to patients?* How was this money "invested" and at what return? Was this investment ever liquidated and where did the money go?

(4) Hospital director stated increased rates were needed due to price increases in payrolls, equipment, utilities and other commodities. These basic costs were included in U.S. Department of Labor statistics under "all items" category—increased approximately 40 per cent from 1960 to 1970. *Hospital rates increased approximately 200 percent during same period, about 5 times as fast as the rate of general "inflation."* Was it due to excessive salaries and fees paid to medical doctors; to excessive remuneration to pathologists; costs for educational expense to medical students, not properly a cost to be borne by patients in price of beds; charges for "research" which is not a responsibility of patients and the inclusion of which in bed charges is manifestly unfair as any medical advance from such "research" would be for the *general good* and not for the good of the *specific* patient who is forced to pay such charges?

(5) What is the annual cost of "research"?

(6) What has this "research" accomplished?

(7) *How much time do individuals engaged in "research" spend on the job?*

(8) As this state facility which pays no taxes is heavily subsidized by those of us who do, why is information as to salaries at professional and administrative levels refused taxpayers? *Has a state facility the right to "classify" such information as secret? Does not the taxpayer have the right to know where his money goes?*

(9) Are pathologists remunerated on a salary basis or on a percent of the "take" as is the case in some hospitals? [$100,000 a year incomes to these individuals has been reported!]

(10) Were any operating figures supplied as to:

   (A) *Actual* cost of bed service, space, housekeeping, meals, heat, light, maintenance, push button bell service?

   (B) Cost of medical training service to students, etc? (Which should be charged to university itself not to patients.)

   (C) Cost of "research"?

   (D) Cost of laboratory service:

      (1) Service to patients?

      (2) Service to "research" and medical students?

(11) *A state facility of this type with revenue exceeding $40,000,000 annually should be strictly accountable to taxpayers* as to its efficiency of operation, sound and competent management, purchasing practices, information as to administrative and professional salaries, organization and control of personnel and work flow. *When such information and accountability is refused or withheld by any state facility it suggests that there is something to hide.*

I do not believe that it is the will or intention of voters and taxpayers in this state to set up and support an academic, autocratic and bureaucratic elite with *no public accountability, exempt such a facility from taxation* and *give them free rein to charge all the traffic will bear* for the services they supply to the taxpayers who make their existence possible.

Rex Dye

Rex Dye Advertising

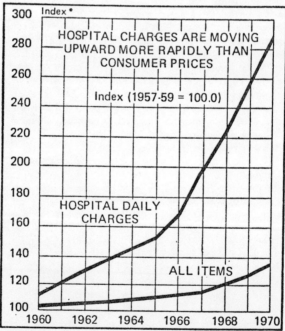

Government statistics indicate your present coverage may be inadequate to meet today's rising costs. That's why you can't afford to be without this low-cost, high-benefits Tax-Free Hospital Benefits Policy.

*Source: United States Department of Labor

None of the regents responded to this memo. Taxpayers and patients who pay the bills are not supposed to ask embarrassing questions!

Hospital patients are charged for training medical students and "research" which are, in theory, for the general good and which by no possible sound reasoning could be justifiably considered as a part of the legitimate expense incurred by the specific patient. Patients are charged for services they never receive, costly equipment they do not use or benefit from, expenses for travel they do not participate in, and costly "public relations" activities that only serve to facilitate the exploitation of the health market.

If hospitals were as efficient in serving patients as they are in collecting money from them no national health crisis would be likely to exist. Let me cite a few incidents appearing in "Action Line" of the *Detroit Free Press*. (In case you have noticed that most of my citations from newspapers are from this outstanding paper, let me say that if I were to attempt to include cases from the press on a national basis it would, I believe, take a set of volumes of encyclopedic size to present them!)

Incident 1: A baby girl was born at Sinai Hospital and had to stay a couple of extra days. Blue Cross did not cover this added expense and the hospital threatened to garnishee the husband's pay because a computer found "no known relationship" between his wife and the baby!

"Action Line" got the hospital and Blue Cross together and found that the baby was "a close relative of the wife" and induced Blue Cross to pay! (Where would they have been without "Action Line"?)

Incident 2: While visiting at Lansing, Michigan, a wife had to go to Sparrow Hospital for emergency eye treatment. They got a bill for pregnancy treatment. The hospital got a collection agency after them!

"Action Line" got a letter of apology, for somebody failed to "feed data to the computer." (The computer is a great asset to a hospital as it can be blamed for errors and overbilling in favor of the hospital if discovered.)

Incident 3: A couple paid the doctor in advance for their daughter's operation. The doctor also collected from Blue Cross and refused to refund prepayment.

"Action Line" got the Consumer Protection Division to have a chat with that doctor. The couple got their refund.

Incident 4: Henry Ford Hospital received an advance payment of $1,273 for projected services. The final total billing was $962.50, the hospital owing the patient $310.50. After four months they could not get the hospital to refund.

"Action Line" got the refund in four minutes! Hospital excuse was misfiling.

Incident 5: Blue Cross covered part of a bill from Mt. Clemens General Hospital. The patient needed an itemized bill in order to collect the balance from another insuror. Instead of helping clear the matter the hospital got a collection agency after her!

"Action Line" got the itemized bill. Hospital spokesman told "Action Line" they sent itemized bills directly to insurance companies and only total bills to individuals!

This type of handling billing keeps the patient from knowing what services he was supposed to have received, prevents him from checking the bill and facilitates overbilling and padding of bills by the hospital.

Incident 6: A five-year-old fell and cut his head. His parents took him to Beaumont General Hospital. He was cared for by an intern. They got a bill from a doctor they had never heard of.

"Action Line" cleared the matter and was told by the claims advisor of the parents' insuring company that about ten percent of the claims it pays are for services not rendered!

Incident 7: A patient was unable to call his wife while at University Hospital as there was only one phone on his floor for 100 patients.

"Action Line" convinced hospital officials, and phones were to be installed when the hospital "comes up with the money" (but they had nearly $2,000,000 of excess funds to "invest" with the university in 1970! Patients or their loved ones are given little consideration!)

Incident 8: A patient had been at University Hospital twice, giving $300 deposits each time, though fully insured. He could not get the money the hospital owed him even after the insurance company had paid the hospital.

"Action Line" got the $600 refund for him!

These eight incidents give only a glimpse of the hospitals' greed for money. Ruth Winter in *How to Reduce Your Medical Bills** says,

---

*Ruth Winter, *How to Reduce Your Medical Bills* (New York: Crown Publishers, Inc., 1970).

"One reason for the variation in charges is evidently how much hospitals are willing to pad your bill." This might account for the fact that some hospitals do not give patients itemized bills. (See Incident 5 above.) She also states a large supplier of pharmaceuticals says that hospitals pay 76 cents for a bottle of 1,000 aspirins and charge 50 cents to one dollar for each tablet given a patient, a gross profit of from $500 to $1000—700 percent to 1,400 percent over cost! Speaking of nonprofit hospitals she writes that they often show a profit and that these profits are used by trustees to visit other states and attend conferences, often nothing more than paid vacations.

I suggest that you get a copy of this book and read it thoughtfully. It will give you an insight into the problem of health care that may not only save you money but give you an understanding of medical care that can protect your health.

I also suggest that you get Senator Edward M. Kennedy's book, *In Critical Condition* and read thoughtfully Chapter I, "Sickness and Bankruptcy," and Chapter VII, "Businessmen or Healers," particularly,*

While I do not feel that federal bureaucracies will solve the hospital/medical problem, this book presents a clear picture of the extent of that problem and its critical state today.

The cost of hospital, surgical, medical and drug care is shared not only by patients and insurance companies but also by new car buyers. Mr. McKenna of the Ford Motor Company was reported as saying that Ford premiums increased from $41.69 *per month* per employee in 1970 to $66.09 in 1972, an increase of 59 percent in less than two years. This cost is a fringe benefit to employees, and in any industry operating for profit must be reflected in the selling price of the product. $793.08 of cost per employee per year must be absorbed by new car prices in Ford Motor sales alone. General Motors, Chrysler and American Motors, of course also have this cost figure which must be included in pricing. When you consider this cost impact of employer-paid medical and hospital insurance at uncontrolled rates on the increased prices of all types of consumer goods, the aggregate retail price increase runs into billions of dollars.

---

*Edward M. Kennedy, *In Critical Condition: The Crisis in America's Health Care* (New York: Pocketbooks, 1973).

It was reported on April 24, 1972, that Michigan's Medicaid program cost nearly $263 million in 1971, $57 million or 28 percent higher than in 1970. HEW statistics showed that hospitals received $98 million of this, a 46 percent increase over 1970, while doctors' fees totaled $31.7 million, a 46 percent increase over 1970.

The following letter to Dolores Katz, medical writer for the *Detroit Free Press,* outlines some of the reasons for exorbitant hospital charges.

Dolores:

Please excuse my rather informal salutation. I cannot reconcile myself to using the semantically meaningless "Ms." (which to me suggests "manuscript") and therefore refrained from using the customary "Dear."

I enjoyed reading your very well-written piece "Michigan Hospitals Can Save $55 Million" in the 12/18/72 *Free Press.* I am sure Dr. Levagood has isolated one very significant factor responsible for excessive hospital costs. There are several other "money wasters" which should be thoroughly checked and would, I believe, result in greatly reducing hospital *charges* as well as real costs. They are:

(1) *Time waiting for finalizing diagnosis*—Three doctors told me that my wife's diagnosis of terminal cancer should have been made at University Hospital in half the time taken, which would cut bed time in half. They also had my assurance that their names would not be disclosed, apparently fearing censure by their "peers" as was the case with Dr. Knowles, now president of the Rockefeller Foundation.

(2) *Hidden costs*—such as "research" and medical student training, not honestly chargeable to the specific patient yet concealed in bed charges without patient's knowledge.

(3) *Monopolistic character*—Doctors send people to hospitals. No truly competitive market exists. People cannot shop for hospital service. Hospitals can and do charge all they can get and sue to the point of bankruptcy those who cannot pay. A program on Channel 4, 12/19/72 at 10 P.M., illustrated this vicious attitude effectively.

(4) *Favored treatment of "V.I.P's"*—Ward patients and insurors pay the way for the affluent. If the influential were billed on a basis comparable to billing to ward patients the charge would be in the neighborhood of $1,000 per day instead of the $102 per day for "plush service" and quarters available at Ford Hospital.

(5) *Excessive salaries and fees*—The medical trust has apparently restricted "output" of M.D.'s by medical colleges far below the need of the nation, particularly as to work in family practice. Outdated teaching of medicine, excessive hospital intern and resident time contribute to high hospital charges. (See Ruth Winter's

book *How to Reduce Your Hospital Bills,* an excellent, thorough and well-documented work published by Crown Publishers; also see the article from the *Northville Record* [December 6, 1972] re Dr. Robert Vitu, president of Michigan Academy of Family Practice in which the statement is made, "Various forms of snobbery, prestige, tradition and inertia seem to be involved on the part of medical educators . . . University of Michigan Medical School appears to be the most dogmatic in ignoring needs of the public—Wayne's doctors seem to be trying almost as hard.")

(6) *Excessive fees and commissions to pathologists*—Some are receiving over $100,000 annually without ordering, performing or interpreting 90 percent of the laboratory tests made according to Ruth Winter in the book previously mentioned. (I suggest you try to learn how and how much pathologists are paid at University Hospital and other state facilities.)

(7) *Secret salaries*—It is hard to believe that salaries paid by taxpayers are concealed, yet such information is denied the public by state universities and hospitals with arrogant disregard of the right citizens have to know how and where our tax money is spent. These academic "elite" apparently regard themselves so far above "ordinary" folks like ourselves that they can ignore with impunity the people who enable them to live very "high on the hog"!

(8) *Withholding excess charges to patients instead of using such "profit" to reduce charges to patients*—University Hospital, Ann Arbor, "Trend Statement 1970" showed approximately $2 million "invested" with University of Michigan. Being a nonprofit, tax-exempt facility of the state this money accumulated by overcharging patients should certainly have been applied to reducing such patient charges. Such action appears to be a violation of the legal and ethical conditions under which a nonprofit organization is granted the right to operate. (This item alone if it had been so applied could have reduced charges to patients by $2 million!) As to *general* price rise being the cause of the gross overcharges by hospitals, this is pure fiction having no basis in fact.

> I am sincerely,
> Rex Dye

Some of the elements in this foregoing outline will be developed more fully in later chapters.

Hospital organizations appear to be efficient and cost conscious in only one phase of their activity; getting all the money that traffic will bear from helpless patients and their families who are completely at the mercy of these institutions.

4

Why Are Hospital/Medical
Insurance Rates Skyrocketing?

During the 1930s I was retained by George Gnau, president and founder of the Detroit Insurance Agency, one of the largest and most efficient in the United States, as research counsel. Study and analysis of insurance fundamentals was essential and I made a thorough study of the subject. When Mr. Gnau sold his interest in the D.I.A. and formed Gnau and Company, I was retained by him in the same capacity. We were also associated in the Insurance Research Bureau. I make this preliminary statement to indicate that my following observations are based on sound experience in this field.

Insurance is a means for the distribution of risk over a broad group in order that those of that group who unfortunately have that risk materialize as actuality may be compensated for their losses.

Insurance rates must be determined by accurate actuarial experience covering frequency of losses with relation to the group insured, and the cost of replacing the values lost or indemnity for the risk assumed. A fair cost, based on bids from a free, competitive market is essential for actuarial experience to be valid.

If you are insured on your home for fire, the frequency and dollar values involved in your area will be one factor in the actuarial basis for determination of rates. The cost of repairing or replacing your house, if fire occurs, will be based on the record of similar costs arrived at by competitive bids in a nonmonopolistic market. These bids will not include items of cost not related to the specific insured hazard, in fact any attempt to include such items would be fraudulent and subject to legal action.

Let us consider the conditions under which hospital insurance rates are based. First, we do not have a competitive market for hospitalization such as we have for fire or automobile hazards. You go to the hospital your doctor suggests. You cannot shop for a price even if you were physically able to. You are at the mercy of a supplier who has no competition and, in effect, has a monopoly, able to charge the patient even to the point of bankrupting him.

Your hospital bill can contain at least two items of "cost" which have no relation whatever to your stay in the hospital; medical student training and "research."

The first of these items, medical student training, is a service to the student, helping him to prepare for a lucrative career in the practice of medicine. The second item, "research," covers activities, at best for the general future good, certainly in no way a proper charge against your period of hospitalization. Yet these two substantial cost factors are included in your bill and become a part of the cost record of insurance companies' actuarial experience! Such cost juggling would be tolerated in no other field of insurance.

I sent the Insurance Bureau of the State of Michigan the following letter enclosing data such as here presented.

Mr. Claude McCann, Director
Health Service Plans Section
Insurance Bureau, Dept. of Commerce
111 N. Hosmer St.
Lansing, Michigan

Dear Mr. McCann:

I appreciate your letter of April 17, 1972 and the April 7th bulletin you enclosed.

I believe the Insurance Bureau in dealing with rate increase demands by Blue Cross should keep in mind:
    I. That rates are based on totally unrealistic charges by hospitals. The daily rate at University Hospital, Ann Arbor (for ward beds), being approximately *three times* that for which far better bed service is available elsewhere.
    II. That the "public representatives" on the Blue Cross Board are

selected from lists of names submitted by hospitals surely not in the public interest!

III. That huge advertising and "public relations" expenditures by Blue Cross designed to create and maintain the illusion that the public is getting insurance protection at a fair price based on actual costs is totally unfair and serves to maintain excessive premium rates.

IV. That bed charges, such as at University Hospital include "hidden costs" such as student training expense and "research" which certainly cannot be considered as legitimate charges to patients hospitalized for specific illnesses. Yet these concealed costs are included in insurance actuarial experience and are passed on to 5,000,000 policy holders, in excessive premiums not based on sound actuarial experience with realistic costs! (And subscribers' own money is spent lavishly in full-page newspaper ads and television in an attempt to defer a day of reckoning!)

V. That a virtual hospital/medical monopoly exists with charges skyrocketing beyond all other prices and that this situation is headed for a public disclosure that will leave major repercussions.

In casualty, fire and auto insurance, insurance rates are based on losses where values involved are subject to accurate determination in a competitive market. In the hospital/medical field values such as bed charges, doctors' fees, laboratory tests and medication are subject to no competitive market or apparently other controls. Hospital charges are increased to include expenditures not properly chargeable to the service actually given.

Blue Cross/Blue Shield seems to be more of a collection agency securing prepayment of excessive charges for the hospital/medical combine than an actual insurance organization operating on a basis of sound risk distribution and true costs of the services for which the policy holder is "insured."

Blue Cross itself has little incentive to investigate cost controls in hospitals, in fact the higher the hospital billing the higher their rates go and the more money they have for high salaries, expense accounts, and heavy advertising and "public relations" spending.

The fact that University Hospital charged three times as much for bed space as far better bed space and service was available for elsewhere, illustrates why Blue Cross asks for rate increases!

It seems to me that, as a matter of public interest, the Insurance Bureau should have the power to investigate the rate structure of hospital insurance and the validity of the charges made by hospitals on which these rates are based. No insurance organization can be financially sound if the risk it insures (whether a car accident, fire loss, other casualty or hospital stay) is subject to unrestrained noncompetitive pricing by those who provide the services covered.

Approval of rate increases by the state is actually, I believe, serving to protect and perpetuate an unsound and uncontrolled situation that is fast becoming critical.

I am,

Sincerely,
Rex Dye

I cannot imagine that a hospital would supply candidates not willing to go along with hospital thinking as against the welfare of policy holders. Is it any wonder that Ford Motor Company reported an increase in premiums of 59 percent in less than two years?

In a thorough analysis of the Blue Cross, *Blue Cross—What Went Wrong?* (prepared by the Health Law Project, University of Pennsylvania, of which Sylvia S. Law was the principal author, Yale University Press, publishers), the failure of this insuring group is brought into sharp focus and reasons based on exhaustive research are given for the failure of this complex to function in the public interest.

This book brings out the fact that Blue Cross is dominated by hospitals; that Blue Cross has no federal supervision and is not regulated in the consumer interest; and that Blue Cross administers Medicare for the Social Security Administration with virtually no supervision or controls.

This book presents examples of serious conflicts of interest such as deposits of millions of dollars in noninterest-bearing accounts with banks having officers and board members on Blue Cross Boards. When we have a prime rate of 10 percent or more on loans of minimum risk, this practice is certainly a windfall to the banks involved and certainly not in the interest of the public who are paying health insurance premiums.

When you realize that over $11 billion is paid to hospitals annually by Blue Cross you will get an idea of the forces involved in the rape of the health market.

This report brings out the fact that the hospitals dominating Blue Cross are organized for "research" and to meet the needs of doctors and "researchers" rather than to meet the needs of the public.

The political and financial relationships between Blue Cross top personnel and our elected officials and heads of health related bureaus at state and national levels should be subject to penetrating investigation and full access to findings by the press.

The huge amount of money spent by Blue Cross in newspaper, television and radio advertising to delude the public into believing they are operating in the public interest should also be brought under control and the advertising content reviewed with relation to the facts of operation.

Federal effort to solve the problem of health insurance cannot hope to be successful unless the real problem of price reduction on health care costs is solved. This cannot be solved without recognition of the fact that a covert monopoly exists in the field nor without full investigation of specific hospitals and their practices by fully competent cost analysts and efficiency engineers.

Actuarial experience taken from inflated hospital billings does not reflect honest real costs of efficient hospitalization for the specific patients and rates based on such experience are not valid.

The *Detroit Free Press* on February 16, 1975, carried a story that Michigan Blue Cross/Blue Shield was asking for another rate increase averaging 23.9%; Blue Cross asking for 22% and Blue Shield for 26.8%. Yet federal and state action to determine the actuarial experience upon which the health insurance rate structure is based is sadly lacking. How much of this "experience" is due to hidden medical student training charges, "research" charges, also hidden bill padding, "profits" by nonprofit hospitals, needless travel expense by hospital officials and related exploitation of the health market is still a secret.

5

Hospitalization at Bargain Rates for the Influential and Other "Public Relations" Activity

Hospitals apparently realize the fact that to maintain their freedom from controls and continue their exploitation of the general public they must have the cooperation and goodwill of the affluent and influential. One of the very effective ploys used is to supply deluxe hospitalization service to such people at what are bargain rates compared to the charges for ward service.

The *Detroit Free Press,* on July 19, 1971, carried a story headed "Hospitals Offer Plush Life," by Susan Holmes, a staff writer. The story told how at "two o'clock sharp" a select group of patients at Henry Ford Hospital were served "tea and crumpets" on monogrammed china from an ornate silver service.

The "ultimate in elegance" at Henry Ford Hospital was described as having a parlor with a bar and remote control color television, a bedroom with rolltop desk, floral wallpaper and special direct-dial telephone which bypassed the hospital switchboard. The suite also had a sofa bed for the convenience of family members who might stay overnight.

The charge for these deluxe quarters, special meals and services was only $102 per day in 1971. Such a suite occupied enough floor area for perhaps 10 or 15 ward beds, which at University Hospital cost $68 per day in the same year, a difference of only $34 per day! Apparently those who enjoy the "plush" life at hospitals do so at the expense of ward patients or ward patients and insurors are being grossly over-charged.

I wrote the *Detroit Free Press* as follows.

Ms. Susan Holmes
The Detroit Free Press
321 W. Lafayette
Detroit, Michigan

Dear Ms. Holmes:

Your story on plush life at hospitals of Monday, 19 July, 1971, illustrates graphically one of the reasons why hospital costs are exorbitant and why hospital insurance rates are climbing.

At University Hospital, Ann Arbor, the charge for a bed in a ward, separated from other beds by a rough canvas pull curtain and occupying space about 7' ✕ 4' costs $55 per day. [In 1970—in 1972 $71 per day and with a 9 percent increase in 1974 to $78 per day!]

The "ultimate in elegance" $102-a-day suite at Ford Hospital with parlor, bar, remote control TV, bedroom, direct-dial switchboard and, of course, special services (at less than twice the cost of a ward bed) would provide room for eight to ten of the ward beds for which the hospital would charge around $500 per day! And, of course, the ward beds provide none of the "luxurious" items you mention which would add substantially to this $500 per day figure for the ward beds.

It would appear from your story that those occupying ward beds are either being grossly overcharged or that those occupying the "ultimate in elegance" are paying far less than they should.

Apparently the ward patients, and/or their insuring companies are paying the major part of the cost of these elegant rooms in excessive charges, while those occupying these rooms are receiving these extra facilities at the expense of those far less able to pay.

If you were to take the time to visit and inspect the $55 per day ward bed areas at University Hospital and compare with the $102-a-day suite you wrote of, I'm sure you would find it difficult to satisfy yourself on why ward space of this character should sell at about *ten times the rate charged for the luxury space!*

I believe even the publicity writers for these hospitals would find it impossible to come up with a believable story to rationalize this disparity.

Sincerely,
Rex Dye

Henry Ford Hospital is not alone in catering to the influential at bargain rates. According to a story in the *Detroit Free Press,* February 24, 1973, by Judith Frutig, a *Free Press* staff writer, St. Joseph Hospital in Pontiac, Michigan, is equally attentive to the needs of the influential.

It was reported that a patient here enjoyed a dinner ordered from room service over a princess telephone in his suite consisting of: Green split pea soup with diced tomato, veal cordon bleu with spiced apple ring, asparagus spears with hollandaise sauce, poppyseed roll with butter and honey, stuffed peach halves a la Cullen (named after the hospital director!) and cream puff a la mode. Of course no such meals would be available to a ward patient!

These quarters and services included: a sleeping room with 19 inch color television, princess telephone, private bath and shower, desk, comfortable chairs, lamps, desk light, deluxe carpeting, wallpaper and drapes.

An adjoining sitting room is provided with desk and highbacked chair, desk lamp, coffee table, hide-a-bed sofa for overnight guests, floor lamp, 19 inch color television, radio and princess telephone.

Additional features included free dictation machine, nearby lounge and game room, free morning and evening newspapers, special visiting hours and courtesy discharge with the bill mailed.

At this time the charge for a ward bed at University Hospital was $71 per day. The charge for the above deluxe treatment was $130 per day. The ward patient got a space of about 4' x 7', enclosed with a rough canvas pull curtain, yet paid over half the price users of this deluxe suite were charged with all its special meals and services, a suite which occupied space equal to ten or more ward beds!

Providence Hospital at Detroit was also reported in 1971 to have deluxe accommodations for the influential at bargain rates, which include remote control television, private princess telephone and other luxury features for $87.50 per day.

Sinai Hospital offered spacious 17' × 16' luxury quarters with private showers, refrigerator and extra sinks for only $91 per day— enough space for about 8 ward beds allowing 114 square feet for a seven-foot aisle in the center of the room for which the charge at University Hospital would have been at least $440 per day!

In fairness, I must state that I do not believe patients occupying such quarters realize that they are objects of "charity" in receiving these bargain rates far below the prices ward patients are forced to pay for bed space, meals and nonmedical service.

Dolores Katz of the *Detroit Free Press* closed an article on luxury suites at hospitals with a short paragraph that expresses a reaction to the foregoing that I believe would be shared by the vast majority of people. She wrote "In a nation where babies are born sick or dead because their mothers received inadequate prenatal care, the picture of a corporate executive having tea and crumpets in his carpeted hospital suite is somehow distasteful."

6

Keeping the Public in Ignorance

In no other major market is the buyer so insulated from information on the product or service it is buying as in the market for health services. In 1971 federal outlays alone for health care were expected to exceed $20 billion for the year. The total national cost of medical care for the fiscal year ending in 1969 reached over $60 billion according to a report of U.S. Department of Health, Education and Welfare of February 27, 1970. This is obviously a huge market, yet practically no "consumers" in this market have any idea of what they are actually paying for. They are trying to buy freedom from pain, avoidance of death, repair of injury, restoration of health—but they cannot know whether a diagnosis is valid, whether the drugs or services prescribed are correct for their troubles or whether the doctor they have gone to is competent or is willing to take time to give a valid opinion. They are unable to shop for competitive prices on services required and often are under dreadful emotional pressures which would make this difficult or impossible even if no monopolistic controls existed.

How many patients can read and understand a doctor's prescription? How many patients can check a hospital bill and have any idea of what laboratory charges and medication mean? How can a patient at a hospital know when he is being overbilled or billed for services not received?

Consider that medical terminology employs a dead language for communication, a language understood (perhaps not fully) only by the initiated medical practitioners who have spent needless years in learning the application of this esoteric means of communication for the medical elite. This terminology, semantically meaningless to the

49

vast majority, serves to keep the market in ignorance of what they get for the money they pay.

This terminology serves not only to impress the market with its assumed "scientific" scholarship and authority and keep that market in ignorance, but also serves to protect its users from their own disastrous mistakes. How can patients or their loved ones know when they are being "taken"?

The "consumer" in the health market must buy on faith and hope under the pressure of desperation and, to date, has been given little or no protection by federal, state or local government.

It seems clear that a defacto monopoly exists. Senator Hart referred some of the material I sent him to the anti-trust division of the Department of Justice, but I have heard no further on possible action at the time this book was written. It is quite possible that the impact of Watergate and related infamous activities have delayed action on this problem.

Secrecy and isolation of the public as to information on hospital/medical affairs is not limited to semantic techniques. The arrogant refusal to divulge vital information is also used to prevent the taxpaying public from learning where their money is going and what they are getting for it.

Secrecy as to salaries paid to professors and administrators of medicine at the University of Michigan, its hospital and other state educational institutions, is withheld from the taxpayer who foots the bill by, in my opinion, a highly questionable legal device called "constitutional autonomy." This device permits universities and university hospitals to operate with no obligation or responsibility to the taxpayer as to their use of taxpayer money.

In December of 1971, Professor Bob F. Repas of Michigan State University dropped a bombshell into the "elite" academic world of Michigan by publishing the "confidential" list of academic salaries paid. Among the highest salaries paid were those of professors and administrators of medicine—$40,000 to $43,000 annually. The publication did not, of course, give any information as to their other income from lucrative private practice, which I have been told some professors of medicine maintain. A letter to Mr. Connors, director of University

Hospital, a facility of the University of Michigan, requesting such information regarding hospital staff was ignored.

The public, insofar as hospital medical costs are concerned, is supposed to pay whatever is charged without asking any questions as to how the charges were determined! The public is to be kept in ignorance of all aspects of health care and cost factors entering into the exorbitant billing. State government officials as well as the regents of our universities (with exception of the two regents previously cited) go along with this policy of secrecy.

I cannot help but wonder how much political pressure and campaign contributions from the medical profession has to do with the reluctance of state and national officials to act to clean house in this area. More detail will be given on the reactions I have had from politicians in a subsequent chapter.

The buyer in the health market may have a Ph.D. in some other specialty, may be a highly informed, well-read and intelligent individual, yet is likely to be a babe in the woods when his health is at stake and must deal with a medical problem.

7

The Problem of Producing Doctors

A major and primary function of state university medical education is to produce physicians qualified to practice. That universities are not functioning properly in this phase of education is recognized by everyone familiar with the health care problem. The problem is not one of student desire and capacity for medical education but one of failure on the part of the "academic elite" in the field of medical education to adjust their thinking to the twentieth century and establish a curriculum and acquire a social and economic viewpoint geared to the needs and problems of today.

In the *Northville Record,* a weekly newspaper in a small Michigan suburb of Detroit, a story under the headline "State Takes a Hard Look at Doctor Shortage" appeared on December 6, 1972. This excellent story brought the basic problem and why that problem exists into clear focus.

It stated that Michigan medical educators had failed to realize that the country is in dire need of doctors who will work with the public and that it is their business to produce such doctors. This was said to be the opinion of Dr. Robert Vitu, a Saginaw physician, president of the Michigan Academy of Family Practice.

The article stated that various forms of snobbery, prestige, tradition and inertia seemed to be involved on the part of medical educators. These medical educators are the people who decide which applying students will be accepted for medical training, what they will be taught and how they will be taught. Their failure to recognize and react to the problems of late twentieth century health serves to accentuate the approaching crisis and contribute to its disastrous effect in the field of health care.

The article stated that the record did not indicate that the medical educators were interested in training doctors for general practice but were more interested in turning out doctors for research and specialized practice, and further, that students were discouraged when they expressed a desire for family practice and told "you'll get over it"! This attitude is certainly against public interest.

The University of Michigan appeared to be the most dogmatic in ignoring the needs of the public for family practitioners, the article continued, with Wayne State University not far behind in this regard.

The Academy for General Practice of which Dr. Vitu is president, urged that Michigan medical schools set up family practice departments so students interested in such practice could be trained for it, but reported that little progress had been made with the medical schools toward this goal, in spite of the fact that numerous students had written Dr. Vitu regarding their desire for family practice.

Dr. Vitu was said to have felt that the outlook for immediate change on the part of medical schools with regard to training for family practice was bleak.

Graduates of osteopathic schools were said to be more inclined to set up practice in communities, and from my own experience osteopathic physicians are, today, more sympathetic, responsive and attentive than the M.D. For example, after a severe bout with the "flu" I was left with loss of equilibrium which was corrected under the care of an osteopath, but a constant ringing in the ears at varied frequencies persisted. My doctor referred me to an osteopathic ear specialist who, after giving several hearing tests and discussing the problem with me at some length, told me that he could do nothing further as the condition appeared to be chronic and did not respond to treatment. The charge for the office visit was $5. Appointments made with this doctor were kept without excessive waiting although there was steady patient traffic.

At the suggestion of friends, I later made appointments with two different M.D. ear specialists. The first "specialist" rushed me through a hearing test. The audiologist, a high-sounding name for a Ph.D. having no M.D. degree, went through the hearing test fast—and then tried to sell me a hearing aid! A hearing aid could in no way serve to correct loss of equilibrium nor act to correct the constant ringing in the ears, and the attempt to sell me a hearing aid seemed to me to be close to malpractice. The charge for the hearing test was $15. The audiologist was more interested in getting the fast $15 and probably a juicy profit on a hearing aid than in my well-being. The second "specialist's" office gave the usual fast hearing test at the exorbitant $15 fee, and, after one hour past my appointment time, I told the receptionist I was leaving and was sorry the doctor could not keep his appointment with me. The doctor did not have the courtesy or consideration for my time to notify me of the delay or to explain it.

The M.D. specialists did not show anywhere near the understanding of my problem shown by the D.O. specialist and charged three times as much for their hearing tests which were not as thorough or time-consuming as the tests given by the D.O.

With increasing awareness on the part of legislators, more funds may be supplied for osteopathic training. This might, to some extent, serve to relieve the doctor shortage.

But the problem of producing doctors rests with university medical schools which seem to be far more concerned with maintaining the shortage of doctors (1) by limiting the number of students accepted for training (2) maintaining outdated curriculums, and (3) their insistence on excessive time requirements to complete training and receive degrees. Much of the college level schooling could be given to intelligent students at the high school level! The time of the student is wasted and the public who pay the bills get little for the price they pay.

In the May-June issue of *The Center Magazine* is an article, "Medicine in China" by Paul T. K. Lin, which should be read and studied by every medical educator, every health insurance executive, every legislator and every doctor in the United States.

The radical advances made in the recruitment of students, in the curriculum and in the placement of graduates from medical schools in China since the Cultural Revolution might well be studied with relation to our own health problems and particularly to solving the problem of the doctor shortage.

The shift in motivation from the dollar income consciousness to social consciousness, from "big doctor" status and prestige to devotion to service in the field of health care, from academic insulation from "ordinary" folks to becoming one with those people would go far to a solution.

Chinese medical students begin clinical work in the latter part of a three-year curriculum. Paramedics, taught to "know what they know" and also "what they do not know" are constantly being upgraded in their training and some finally enter medical schools.

Previously, medical research which focused on rare esoteric cases which could bring national or international fame by brilliant discovery has shifted in focus to most prevalent diseases and egotistical motivation replaced by motivation to service.

The foregoing only highlights elements dealing primarily with producing doctors. The article gives information on health care delivery and costs in Communist China which might well be studied by the health care industry in capitalistic America!

Our "doctor shortage" appears to be artificial and contrived due to the failure of medical educators to recognize their obligation to society to train healers and to open the door to medical training to all students qualified for such training.

8

Political Aspects of the Problem

To understand, in part, the political involvement of hospital/medical interests in state and federal government it is necessary to become involved in trying to secure information and get constructive corrective action initiated from governmental bodies. Keeping in mind the fact that you are questioning the motivations and methods of a $63 billion "health care" industry (in 1969), and probably exceeding $70 billion today, the financial and political power of this group is apparent.

I wrote Governor Milliken of Michigan in 1971, sending a photostat of the memo I had sent to University Hospital at Ann Arbor in 1970 and which was printed in chapter two of this book. I also enclosed a photostat of the letter received from Mr. Zugich which stated the communication was one of the "most constructive letters which could have been received by management."

The response I got from the governor, typically a political piece of buckpassing, follows:

Dear Mr. Dye:
Thank you for your letter of March 1, 1971, and the enclosed memorandum regarding the operation of the University Hospital, University of Michigan Medical Center, Ann Arbor, Michigan.

I share your concern for the high cost of health care, its quality and the need to assure proper utilization of services and ancillary resources. Your comments in this regard are both interesting and provocative.

On the other hand, information provided me indicates that the University Hospital and its medical staff justify the outstanding reputation they have earned in the many years of providing comprehensive high quality service to the citizens of this state. The University Hospital, under new administration, is currently reorganizing as part of its continuing effort to further improve its facilities and services.

I am forwarding a copy of your letter to Mr. Edward J. Connors, director, University Hospital, so that he may have the opportunity to review your comments. I'm sure that you will hear from him soon.

Thank you for bringing this matter to my attention.

Kind personal regards.

> Sincerely,
> Governor William G. Milliken

He "shared my concern" and my comments were "interesting and provocative"—but he passed the buck to Mr. Connors, the hospital director who, in 1974, was found to have overbilled $8,000 in travel expenses since 1971, about the time I wrote the governor. You will note that the governor stated in the above letter that he had been informed that University Hospital and staff justified their "outstanding reputation." He did not, however, say where this information came from. Had he acted to have this state facility investigated at the time of my letter he might have discovered the overbilling before it amounted to $8,000 and that later cost Mr. Connors his $45,000-a-year job.

In response to the governor's letter I wrote as follows:

Dear Governor:

I greatly appreciate your letter of March 23, 1971, relative to the University Hospital.

I sent the "memo" you received to Mr. Connors, director of the hospital, in September of 1970, and received a letter from his office (copy herewith) recognizing the validity of the data sent.

I have no reason to question Mr. Connors' intent or ability to reorganize this institution, but unless he has support from high enough levels to overcome the set patterns, policies and administrative inadequacies of the medical academic fraternity whose decisions govern operation, I do not see how he or any director can overcome the conditions that existed in 1970.

Your support of his effort to reorganize this institution, would, in my opinion, be sound action in the public interest.

The accompanying comparative analysis of bed costs has, I believe, a direct bearing on requests by insuring institutions such as Blue Cross, for higher rates.

This comparative data is an actual case record based on facts which any cost analyst could not ignore. And this relates to only one hospital. What must be the effect on hospital insurance actuarial experience faced with such charges beyond any real cost?

Millions of Michigan taxpayers are faced with this problem and in my opinion, when you consider the millions of dollars involved, this is a public issue of first importance.

Sincerely,
Rex Dye

The governor did not bother to reply to this letter, but did some months later recommend that the state develop "standards and enforcement mechanisms" relating to the quality and cost of health care. A "Technical Work Group on Health Care Costs" was established and two years later (!) came up with a "report": "Rising Medical Costs in Michigan"—547 pages of fine print, including 35 pages of references also in fine print, to show how hard the "Work Group" had worked.

The report is an excellent example of the bureaucratic approach to any problem and an outstanding example of the application of Parkinson's "Law of Delay," of creating the impression of action without acting, of creating the atmosphere of work done yet without accomplishment.

One competent efficiency engineer sent in to University Hospital with full powers to investigate could have prepared a report that might well have revolutionized hospital management and cut costs in terms of charges to patients and insurors in half, provided, of course, that their report was acted on and publicized.

I wrote the governor again, calling attention to the critical nature of the situation.

Dear Governor:
Reference my letter to you of May 24, 1971, and your direction to state health and insurance officials to develop a program for hospital/doctor charges regulation, please send me names of those in charge of this action so that I may send them pertinent data.

It is interesting to note that the "public representatives" on Blue Cross Boards are elected by the Blue Cross Board *from lists submitted by participating hospitals* according to data I've received from Senator Hart—one of the few politicians who seem interested in cleaning up this situation.

It is highly unlikely that hospitals would submit names of those who would not support excessive hospital/medical charges and, to paraphrase a statement by one of the witnesses before Senator Hart's committee, "is like expecting the Mafia to direct the Justice Department."

Over 5,000,000 Michigan residents pay premiums to Blue Cross and those premiums are largely based on excessive charges by hospitals (among which the University Hospital, *a state-owned facility, and example setter,* is a prime example).

When a full disclosure of the situation reaches the public, and I feel this surely will happen, public resentment will make this one of the hottest questions confronting the state.

Sincerely,
Rex Dye

Again I received no response. Apparently the governor did not want to be bothered.

Six months later I wrote again.

Dear Governor:

I am enclosing a preliminary analysis chart and some further informative reproductions of press clippings bearing on the hospital/medical combine and soaring costs far above rises on all other items.

Last year you directed state health and insurance officials to develop a program for regulating hospital and doctor charges. Has any action been taken by these people?

The 1970 trend statement of University Hospital showed $2,000,000 "invested" with University of Michigan. How "invested" and at what rate of return? Why was this "profit" not used to cut costs to patients?

What are the salaries paid to professors and administrators of medicine at University Hospital? (Also, at University of Michigan?) I wrote University Hospital asking for this information but it was not supplied. Are these people, heavily subsidized by taxpayers, allowed to withhold such information? Or are we taxpayers supposed to just give them a blank check? Why should these costs which boost taxes be concealed from the public?

The influence exerted by the hospital/medical combine on corrective action and controls by state authorities must be terrific to have permitted a situation such as exists to develop, or our "public servants" have given very little attention to a monopolistic activity extracting hundreds of millions of dollars from the Michigan "health market" annually.

I believe you will find the enclosed material interesting and well worth thoughtful consideration and I believe the problem involved is sufficiently serious to warrant top priority treatment by those in a position to initiate and enforce corrective action.

I am sincerely,
Rex Dye

The governor did not see fit to respond to this communication or get answers to the questions raised. After an interval of several months I wrote the governor again, and again I received no reply.

Dear Governor:

In an article by Robert H. Longstaff in the *Washtenaw News Review* you were reported to have stated that public confidence and faith in public officials must be restored if government is to work as it should and further, that an "updating" of the code of ethics for public officials is in order.

I am enclosing a copy of a letter to you dated March 27, 1972, asking eight questions to which every taxpayer and voter in the state is entitled to have honest answers. Requests to other public officials for such answers have not been forthcoming.

How could one have any confidence or faith in public officials who ignore such fully justified requests for information?

Failure to supply such information implies that there must be something to hide and also a contemptuous disregard of the public which pays their salaries!

As to "updating" the code of ethics for public servants, isn't a return to old-fashioned morality and honesty the real answer to this problem? I have observed that the term "politician" is rapidly becoming synonymous with the term "crook" in the minds of many people and even among some of my clients who are in the upper-income brackets.

I have the feeling that you, however, are a man of integrity with an in-grained idealism which may make it difficult for you to deal objectively with the self-serving and devious political and academic influences brought to bear on your office.

I am preparing a series of news releases to be sent to 300 Michigan daily and weekly papers dealing with the hospital/medical situation and would like answers to the questions raised in my letter to you of March 27, 1972. If state-owned facilities are authorized to classify such information as "secret" like the "Pentagon papers" I would like to be so informed.

Sincerely,
Rex Dye

So much for the action of the governor of the state of Michigan to correct the exploitation of Michigan's health market. I suspect that the interests of the financially and politically powerful hospital/medical forces in the state cause more concern in high places at Lansing than does the interests of and welfare of the state's citizens.

The state legislature and other state offices are of course targets for influence and a legislator or officeholder is likely to think twice before antagonizing such powerful political forces.

I wrote state Representative Clifford Smart requesting information as follows:

Dear Mr. Smart:

As you represent House District #60, my home area, I am enclosing a memo regarding conditions I experienced at University Hospital which I feel need correction.

In this connection, could you answer these questions for me?

(1) Does University Hospital pay any taxes to the state?

(2) Do they make financial reports of their operation and, if so, can you supply a current copy?

(3) Where does control of this institution rest, the level of authority above that of director?

Your interest will be appreciated.

Sincerely,
Rex Dye

He referred my letter to Mr. Bennett, legislative analyst of the Republican office, House of Representatives at Lansing, who responded with the following letter.

Dear Mr. Dye:

I have been able to obtain the following information in response to your letter of February 18, 1971.

1. The University Hospital is a non-profit institution and does not pay taxes.

2. Enclosed you will the University Hospital Trend Statement of Operations.

3. The order of control runs from Hospital Director, E. J. Connors, to the Academic Vice-President of the University to the President of the University to the elected Board of Regents of the University and ultimately to the people.

If you have any other questions or if I can be of any further help, please feel free to contact me.

Very truly yours,
Allen M. Bennett

I wrote Representative Smart as follows:

Dear Mr. Smart:

Thank you for having Mr. Bennett prepare and send to me the data on University Hospital.

I am enclosing a short summary of revenues and costs of hospital operation based on number of beds (which indicates basic capacity) and number of employees which I believe you will find of interest.

It seems to me that this institution is being operated as a service to medical students and doctors rather than as a service to the people of the state. Primary emphasis certainly should be placed on service to patients. (See "excessive bed time" and "lack of supervision" pages two and three of memo sent you.)

The excessive charges made as illustrated in accompanying comparisons amply show why medical insurance rates are soaring. People with insurance disregard the outrageous billing of hospitals feeling that their insurance is taking care of it so, "so what." Others often under the heavy emotional strain of grief and tragic illness are in no mental or emotional condition to consider costs and so submit without question to these excessive charges.

My wife died August 14 of last year at Beverly Manor Convalescent Home, cited as an example of what accommodations are available at ⅓ the cost of University Hospital bed charges. Prior to her stay at Beverly Manor she was a patient at University Hospital as noted in the memo case record sent you. I believe she was kept in this unpleasant environment at least twice as long as would have been necessary under efficient hospital management—giving us many more hours together in a clean, pleasant environment only five minutes from our home.

I believe this whole hospital/medical insurance situation is going to explode on a national scale and feel that every effort should be made by those who represent the public to uncover the cause of existing conditions and take corrective action.

Sincerely,
Rex Dye

I received no response to this letter and later, in response to an acknowledgment of a questionnaire from Representative Smart, wrote him this letter.

Dear Mr. Smart:

Glad to get your form letter of March '72. I am in hearty accord with your House Bill 5582 on tax relief to property owners and believe that some action along this line is imperative. I am enclosing a memo bearing on the subject.

With further regard to hospital costs, about which I have previously written you, I am enclosing a preliminary analysis chart and some added data on the subject which has a bearing on this extremely serious and immediate problem. You will find this merits thoughtful study, I believe.

I would like to know salaries paid to professors and administrators of medicine at University Hospital (also at U. of M.). I wrote the hospital asking for this but did not get it! As this is a state facility paying no taxes and so heavily subsidized by those who do, I feel this information should be available to all taxpayers in the state. The state should have no "classified" secret payrolls!

Sincerely,
Rex Dye

I received no reply to this and I was apparently touching a very sensitive area in the last paragraph of this letter! Some months later I wrote Representative Smart again.

Dear Mr. Smart:

Are state facilities authorized to keep salaries paid a secret from the public, from taxpayers who, after all, are the people who come up with the money to pay those salaries? Do you, as a state representative from my district feel that taxpayers have no right to know who gets their money and how much they get? I am sure your answer will be that we DO have this right.

As this fundamental right has been denied me, will you please exercise your good offices to see that this information is forthcoming? (See exhibits A-B-C-D-E herewith.)

Also, do you feel that it is right for hospitals to force the average patient or his insuror to subsidize the cost of deluxe quarters and service to the affluent? Is not this an indirect bribe to those with money to influence their attitudes on hospital legislation and controls? (See exhibit F.)

It is my intention to prepare a series of news releases bearing on these questions to be sent to all newspapers in Michigan. Your position on these questions will be valued.

Sincerely,
Rex Dye

Apparently the questions asked were too hot for Representative Smart to handle and no response was received in answer to this letter.

I wrote to Senator Zollar, enclosing the memo to University Hospital and again enclosing a copy of the letter from Mr. Zugich. The two letters follow:

Dear Sir:

I am enclosing a memo and case data which, in view of your inquiry regarding Medicare and Medicaid payments may be of interest.

Hospital charges appear to me to be excessive, contributing heartily to inflated insurance rates.

It seems strange to me that hospitalization insurance organizations apparently take no action to investigate and curb excessive hospital charges. An investigation of relationships between hospital and insurance administrations might be illuminating.

Sincerely,
Rex Dye

Dear Sir:
With further regard to my letter of 9/3/70, with enclosures relating to University Hospital, Ann Arbor, and its bearing on Medicare and Medicaid payments in the state, I am enclosing copy of a letter received from this hospital which acknowledges the validity of the data sent you and indicates that "corrective action is under way."

Payments made under Medicare and Medicaid *must* reflect charges made by hospitals and the medical fraternity. If a venerable institution such as University Hospital can deteriorate to an extent where apparently drastic reorganization is indicated, what must be the conditions existing in the institutions not so much in the public eye? And what is the cost to Michigan taxpayers and the state?

Sincerely,
Rex Dye

The response from the senator follows:

Dear Mr. Dye:
This is to acknowledge your letter of September 3 and October 2nd.

Please be advised that we are looking into this matter. As you know, an extensive investigation is underway concerning Medicare and Medicaid payments and also hospital costs.

We greatly appreciate having the material you sent to add to our files.

Sincerely,
Charles Zollar

This reply is typical "appreciation" and little else. I wrote again and received no reply.

Dear Senator:
With further regard to the subject matter of my letter of Sept. 3, 1970 and of Oct. 2, 1970, regarding hospital/medical costs and payments made under Medicaid and Medicare plans, I am enclosing a preliminary analysis chart and some added data that may be of interest to you.

Your letter to me of Nov. 6, 1970 was very welcome as it indicated an approach to this problem as did the news item stating you had turned your files over to Attorney General Kelley.

I have heard no more about the grand jury action except the one doctor who had billed Medicare over $100,000 for his services in one year. He must have handled something like 10,000 office calls at $10 per call to do this! Allowing him 300 working days this would average out about 33 patients per day or about 20 minutes per patient from 8 A.M. to 6 P.M. and a short lunch period!

Sincerely,
Rex Dye

I received a mailing from state senator Carl Pursell detailing his accomplishments as a "freshman" senator. I wrote him this letter.

Dear Senator:

I was interested to see your bulletin on record re: bills sponsored by you but was surprised to see no action on what is, I believe, one of the most serious and immediate questions facing the voters of Michigan—the astronomical increase in hospital/medical charges. This situation is vitally significant to every voter in the two counties you serve.

They are either paying excessive insurance rates on hospital/medical coverage or are forced to pay excessive charges to hospitals out of savings or income. This situation is so serious and so immediate that insuring organizations are in jeopardy as the result of fantastic billing by hospitals without relation to *real* costs under efficient management.

I am enclosing a preliminary analysis chart and data which I believe warrants thoughtful study and action. I am looking forward to hearing from you.

Sincerely,
Rex Dye

He replied as follows:

Dear Mr. Dye:

Thank you for sending your very detailed and extensive recommendations regarding our continuing problem of increased hospital charges.

We are now reviewing your material to evaluate the possibility of legislative action.

If you would care to forward us your home address I would be more than happy to consult with the senator from your district on this matter.

Sincerely,
Carl D. Pursell

My home address was engraved on my letterhead and on my envelope, but the senator apparently failed to notice this fact.

I wrote Senator Pursell later asking some critical questions. The letter follows:

Dear Senator Pursell:
Are state facilities authorized to keep salaries paid a secret from the public, from taxpayers who, after all, are the people who come up with the money to pay those salaries? Do you, as a state senator from my district feel that taxpayers have no right to know who gets their money and how much they get? I am sure your answer will be that we *do* have this right.

As this fundamental right has been denied me, will you please exercise your good offices to see that this information is forthcoming? (See A-B-C-D-E herewith.)

Also, do you feel that it is right for hospitals to force the average patient or his insuror to subsidize the cost of deluxe quarters and service to the affluent? Is not this an indirect bribe to those with money to influence their attitudes on   hospital legislation and controls? (See Exhibit F.)

It is my intention to prepare a series of news releases bearing on these questions to be sent to all newspapers in Michigan. Your position on these questions will be valued.

Sincerely,
Rex Dye

No response was had to this letter. The senator apparently had no desire to get involved in any way with the hospital/medical interests or the activity of hospitals supplying luxury service to the affluent and influential at bargain rates.

In an attempt to get action from the attorney general's office of the state of Michigan I wrote Attorney General Kelley and enclosed data such as has been given in previous chapters of this book as follows:

Dear Sir:
With regard to the state investigation of Blue Cross and Blue Shield activities and related grand jury procedure, I am of the opinion that investigation should extend into the area of hospital charges and procedures as evidenced by accompanying data and case record.

Hospitals are apparently operating under a virtual monopoly accepted and approved by insurance company administrators, with price fixing that appears to have little relation to real costs under efficient management and which appears to me to be against public interest. The effect on insurance rates is obvious.

I am,

Sincerely,
Rex Dye

I received no response and wrote again enclosing a copy of the letter from Mr. Zugich of the University Hospital which appears in chapter 2 herein.

Dear Mr. Kelley:
The enclosed copy of a letter from University Hospital, Ann Arbor, is in response to a letter and memorandum sent them, copy of which I sent you on September 3, 1970.

This letter confirms the validity of statements made in this memorandum and indicates that corrective action is being taken.

It is my opinion that conditions outlined in my statement (mailed you) are general, not confined to University Hospital, Ann Arbor. The "pocket book" impact on citizens of the state of Michigan with reference to soaring medical/hospital costs and corresponding increases in insurance premium rates is obvious.

I understand that Blue Cross/Blue Shield alone have around 5,000,000 policy holders in the state, What would be the total number of medical/hospital citizens in the state forced to pay excessive charges due to hospital inefficiency or mismanagement? What would this cost to taxpayers amount to in dollars?

I feel that state action to bring hospitals under effective control as to service and charges is vitally needed if public protection through the existing insurance structure, already in jeopardy, is not to be destroyed.

Sincerely,
Rex Dye

Again I received no reply and about two years later wrote the attorney general as follows:

Dear Mr. Kelley:
Do state facilities have a legal right to withhold information on salaries paid to their employees from the taxpaying and voting public? If they have such a right, under what authority is it based? (Exhibit A.)

Does a state facility organized as a nonprofit institution, paying no taxes and therefore heavily subsidized by those of us who *do,* have a legal right to retain surplus revenue or profit and invest it instead of using that profit to reduce cost of service to patients? (Exhibit B.)

Do hospitals have a legal right to force average patients to subsidize the affluent? (Exhibit C.)

The hospital/medical combine appears to enjoy a monopoly position which enables them not only to exploit a virtually helpless and noncompetitive heath market but also to keep the public from gaining any information on its cost and pricing practice even in state facilities.

As 5,000,000 residents of Michigan are paying excessive health insurance premiums to Blue Cross/Blue Shield alone, the impact on the taxpayer's pocketbook is obvious.

Your response to the foregoing would be greatly appreciated and I will be glad to send you further data if it would be of interest. (Senator Hart wrote me that he had forwarded some of the data sent him to the Department of Justice for consideration.)

I am sincerely,
Rex Dye

This letter was referred to Mrs. Maxine Virtue of the attorney general's staff for reply. Her letter follows:

Dear Mr. Dye:

Your letter of January 8 asking several questions has been referred to undersigned.

This office is unable to entertain requests for opinions from private citizens. For your information, however, you will be interested to know that the extent to which state facilities, such as universities, have a right to withhold information on salaries paid to their employees is now in litigation. It is not a simple question since the universities enjoy constitutional autonomy, and since employees are entitled to have legal protection with respect to certain information contained in their personnel files.

With respect to the accounting requirement applicable to medical care corporations, those corporations are audited by state and federal agencies, and their accounting practices are under the statutory provision of the Commissioner of Insurance, to whom we are forwarding the information you made available.

Thank you for your interest and information.

Yours sincerely,
Frank J. Kelley
Attorney General
(Mrs.) Maxine Boord Virtue
Assistant Attorney General

You will note in the above letter that some state facilities are able to conceal from taxpayers where their money goes, establishing a secrecy system certainly not in the public interest. I wrote Mrs. Virtue the following letter.

Dear Mrs. Virtue:
I was glad to receive your letter of 3/2/73 today, particularly in view of the fact that some state officials simply ignore requests for information.

I realize that your office should not give legal opinions to private citizens. My interest goes beyond the point of a private citizen as such to the area of public interest and I strongly feel that the public interest is being exploited for the benefit of a monopolistic "elite" and that such exploitation is not in the public interest.

While universities may enjoy constitutional autonomy we should not forget the fact that, due to their tax-free status they are heavily subsidized by Michigan taxpayers, and that taxpayers certainly have an inviolable right to know who gets their money, how much they are paid and what they get in return for the salaries paid.

Information of a personal lawful nature might legitimately be withheld but certainly not salaries—any more than the salary paid the president of the U.S. or our governor.

It seems to me that the state would have no sound legal basis under which a constitutional autonomy could be established which denied taxpayers the right to know who they were paying and how much. If this could be legally done for a university or hospital why not for any other state agency such as the highway department, etc.? Set them all up as "constitutional autonomies"?

I read that a University of Michigan student group was starting suit against the university on the salary and other questions and will be greatly interested in the result. Was this the litigation you referred to?

Thank you for your letter and for referring data to Mr. Van Hooser.

Sincerely,
Rex Dye

I have heard nothing further from the attorney general's office.

After I learned of the hearings before Senator Philip A. Hart before the Senate Trust and Antimonopoly Committee on the subject of hospital/medical conditions and costs I wrote the following letter:

Dear Senator Hart:
Your investigation of Blue Cross may well be one of the most important actions in the public interest to occur in many years if thoroughly carried out and fully publicized.

In my opinion, no such investigation can dig out all the facts without an equally thorough investigation of hospitals involved. There must be "understandings" between members of the medical profession in both insurance organizations and in hospitals to allow the situation which exists.

I am enclosing a memo outlining conditions I experienced at University Hospital, Ann Arbor, which I believe you will find revealing. It is my opinion that this institution is *overcharging* for beds alone at the rate of over *$20,000,000 per year*.

This is supported by data contained in accompanying memo and can be easily documented for investigation.

I understand that in *your* state and *mine*, Michigan alone around 5,000,000 people have Blue Cross coverage. Why does Blue Cross stand still for the outrageous charges made by hospitals? It seems to me that solutions to soaring insurance costs may well rest in getting answers to this question.

If University Hospital can overcharge at the rate of $20,000,000 a year on beds alone, what must be the "take" of all hospitals in Michigan annually?

I have the feeling that this question is one of national importance as millions of dollars and thousands of voters are involved.

I hope your investigation gets at the facts . . . that these facts are given to the public . . . and that action is taken to curb the avarice and incompetence that exists in this field.

Sincerely,
Rex Dye

Senator Hart responded as follows:

Dear Mr. Dye:
Your letter is only one of many I have received with respect to the continuous rise in Blue Cross insurance premiums. As a result of such letters and testimony presented during hearings held last year on hospital costs, this subcommittee held hearings in January on Blue Cross plans. Many abuses were brought out at that time.

National health insurance may be the only answer. If it is, then we must be careful that effective controls are part of such a program. In this connection, I am enclosing several statements I have made which you may wish to read.

Sincerely,
Philip A. Hart

The statements he enclosed with his letter included the fact that of $63 billion Americans paid for health care in 1969, almost one-third of it went to hospitals; that our dismal record in health care has been a better-kept secret than many less important facts by the CIA; that competition did not exist in this market; that the patient was not an informed consumer, could not shop for prices and was at the mercy of doctors and hospitals, not only as to care received, but also as to costs. He cited Dr. John Knowles to the effect that cost per patient per day would be $1,000 by 1980, and this is only 26 years away!

His suggestions for reducing hospital costs included eliminating contracts with pathologists whereby they frequently get one-third of laboratory income.

Pathologists in two-thirds of our hospitals were reported to be paid about one-third of the laboratory "take," some pathologists getting annual incomes of $300,000, with annual incomes of $150,000 being not uncommon.

He brought out the fact that the sick are paying for the education of interns, nurses, residents and paramedical personnel at hospitals in spite of the fact that taxpayers support college programs and medical schools. Major teaching hospitals were said to charge as much as $35 per day to the patient for such education.

The relation of hospital to Blue Cross insuring organizations was illustrated by the fact that American Hospital Association owned the Blue Cross emblem until 1972 and that its use by a Blue Cross plan was conditional upon meeting certain requirements of the A.H.A. and that A.H.A. had authority to revoke the license at any time and so put a specific Blue Cross unit out of business!

The ownership of the Blue Cross emblem was transferred to the Blue Cross Association (national) effective June 30, 1972, by the American Hospital Association. A close relationship between A.H.A. and B.C.A. is maintained by a joint committee.

The senator remarked that this raised some interesting antitrust questions.

Apparently the American Hospital Association also subsidizes hospital directors. The *Washtenaw News Review* in October of 1974 reported that Edward J. Connors, director of University Hospital at Ann Arbor, Michigan, charged with felonies by the state attorney general's office, served as a consultant to the association. Connor's remuneration from the association as a consultant (in addition to his $45,000-a-year salary from University Hospital) was not reported.

The fact that hospital trustees and administrators served on the 75 Blue Cross boards across the nation was also mentioned by Hart as raising the question of conflict of interest.

The senator stated that, while consumers assume that insurance companies, acting as their purchasing agents, exercised proper care in paying hospital bills, such is not the case. Cases were on record where patients were billed for medication and treatment not received, yet the insurance company paid, *even over the patient's protests*!

In response to Senator Hart's letter with its enclosure, I wrote this letter:

Dear Senator Hart:

I was glad to receive your letter of April 5th with enclosures, which I found interesting. They cover the general conditions existing and point to the serious need for radical corrective action.

The University Hospital at Ann Arbor is a state-owned institution, paying no taxes and free from many of the expenses of private enterprise. This institution should set an example of how a hospital can be run with greatly reduced bed time, fewer needless "lab" charges and at about ⅓ the daily rate per bed they are charging.

Such an example by a state-operated facility would set standards by which other hospital operations could be judged and to which they would be forced to conform.

Instead of setting such an example, this institution is a prime example of most of the flagrant abuses which are costing the voters in the state alone millions of dollars a year in excessive charges having no relationship to honest and legitimate costs. This state-owned facility sets an example to other hospitals of how to gouge the public, keep patients in beds much longer than efficient operation would make necessary, create an artificial "shortage" of bed space and get by with lowest standards of service to patients.

Similar action by any group other than the organized hospital/medical combine would bring a deluge of investigations, antitrust suits and actions by Better Business Bureaus.

The University Hospital represents the state of Michigan in the hospital world—and it is not, in my opinion, a type of representation the state should be proud of!

Specific action to correct these conditions should be taken by representatives of the people of the state, for the state itself, through its elected officials; its board of regents, president of the university, and academic vice-president of the university, is responsible for the policies and management of this facility.

Sincerely,
Rex Dye

I received this letter from the senator in reply. The letter to Mr. Bennett he refers to appears later herein in connection with the reactions of state politicians and bureaucrats.

Dear Mr. Dye:
Many thanks for your views and also for forwarding me a copy of your letter to Mr. Bennett. I appreciate your bringing your personal experience to my attention and will certainly continue in my efforts to find some way to curb the abuses presently being perpetrated in the health care field. In the meantime, I am enclosing a copy of this subcommittee's hearing record on Blue Cross which you may wish to read.

Sincerely,
Philip A. Hart

I later wrote Senator Hart suggesting specific and public investigation of specific hospitals as follows:

Dear Senator:
Regarding your letter of August 9, 1971, and enclosures (which I have gone over with great interest) it seems to me that in order to achieve substantial corrective action, the public must be made aware of abuses existing and specific action taken to confront the hospital/medical combine with an aroused public opinion.

Five million people in the state are paying hospital insurance to Blue Cross alone unaware of the fact that hospitals select lists of names from which the Blue Cross elects "public" representatives. It is highly unlikely that hospitals would submit names of individuals they could not depend on to go along with the pricing control of the combine. There appears to be a covert agreement to maintain price levels and discourage competition which appears to be a combination in restraint of trade, perhaps warranting some phase of antitrust action.

The fact that, in Michigan, hospitals submit names to be "elected" to the Blue Cross Board leads me to paraphrase Dr. Archambault on page 164 of your Jan. 26, 27 and 28, 1971 hearings, "like accepting candidates selected by the Mafia to sit in judgment on the Justice Department."

It seems to me that a specific and public investigation of University Hospital at Ann Arbor could bring this whole issue to a head and result in overall corrective action. Typical subjects for investigation would include comparative analysis of costs going into bed charges, costs of laboratory service, "investments" with the University of Michigan of $2,000,000, salary levels, individuals selected by the hospital as candidates to Blue Cross Board, possible conflicts of interest, amounts improperly charged to patients and insurors resulting from costs of education of medical students, free space and services to university personnel, etc.

As this is a state-owned institution, it should be a model of how a hospital should and can be run. They pay no taxes and are a "not for profit" organization. Yet their charges are as high or higher than other hospitals, and they have $2,000,000 to "invest" with the University of Michigan. Apparently the board of regents pays little attention to hospital operation.

In fact, it seems to me that doctors and publicity men have done a very effective job on the political representatives of the public at large—to a degree where the hospital/medical trust can suppress undesirable news and largely exempt themselves from any proper controls which would apply in other fields.

It is my belief that this situation will become one of the most serious public issues.

I am sincerely,
Rex Dye

The senator acknowledged this with the following letter:

Dear Mr. Dye:
Thank you for your most recent letter with respect to possible antitrust violations in the physician-hospital-medical insurance combine. I have taken the liberty of forwarding a copy of your letter to the Antitrust Division of the Department of Justice for their views regarding your charges. As soon as I receive a reply, I will write you again.

Sincerely,
Philip A. Hart

My reply follows:

Dear Senator:
I was glad to receive your letter of November 11th and to learn you had forwarded a copy of my letter of September 28th to the Antitrust Division of the Department of Justice.

Their reaction will be of interest to me.

Also, has any action been taken as the result of your committee hearings earlier this year?

I am enclosing some additional material which may be helpful.

Sincerely,
Rex Dye

Not hearing from the senator as any reaction from the Department of Justice I wrote again.

Dear Senator:

As I have not had a reply to my letter to you of March 23, 1972, I am writing again and enclosing some further data on hospital/medical abuses.

In your letter to me of November 11, 1971, you mentioned that you had forwarded copies of my letter of September 28, 1971, to the Department of Justice for consideration. Have you had any response on this? In this connection, the chart I sent you might be of interest. Will send you another copy if you wish.

I am also wondering if there has been any corrective action as the result of your committee hearings, or if the hospital/medical people have been able to exert enough "influence" to prevent any such action. As this field involves hundreds of millions of dollars annually, I realize that heavy pressures can be brought to bear to prevent investigation and corrective action.

Sincerely,
Rex Dye

Six months elapsed with no reply to this letter so I wrote the senator again.

Dear Senator Hart:

You will no doubt recall our previous correspondence regarding the hospital/medical situation and material I sent you, some of which I believe you forwarded to the Antitrust Division of the Department of Justice.

I am enclosing some additional items bearing on this subject which I hope you will find of interest.

It is shocking to me that this monopolistic segment of our population is able to prevent any effective investigation of the activities of members, conceal information from the taxpayers who subsidize their salaries, price their services without regard to real costs or the public interest in complete disregard of price controls and are able to completely insulate themselves from effective state or federal investigation or control.

It seems to me that, much as I dislike the idea of socialized medicine under government control, that the hospital/medical combine will bring this about as the result of their conscienceless exploitation of the health market.

Looking forward to hearing from you as to any further action in this field.

I am sincerely,
Rex Dye

I have received no reply on this and I am inclined to believe that the Washington governmental bodies, elective and bureaucratic, have been so involved in Watergate reactions, repercussions and reprehensibility that little action to correct the abuse of the public by the giant health care industry can be expected and until the air has cleared!

I wrote Martha W. Griffiths of the House of Representatives at Washington. My letter follows:

Dear Mrs. Griffiths:
I am enclosing data on the hospital/medical situation which I believe warrants action on the national as well as the state level.

My deep interest in this problem arose from a disturbing experience at University Hospital while my wife, who died in 1970 of terminal cancer, was a patient there. The "memo" to the hospital outlines this experience and the response to this communication by the hospital indicates agreement with my findings.

I believe a very serious situation exists and would greatly appreciate your views on this as well as any corrective action you may initiate or support.

Sincerely,
Rex Dye

Her reply showed recognition of the problem and outlined features of the Griffiths' Health Security Act. H.R. 22, of which she was chief sponsor. Her comments on University Hospital which should be a model for hospital operation in the state are interesting.

Dear Mr. Dye:
Thank you for your letter and associated documents regarding the costs of hospitalization at the University Hospital in Ann Arbor. You cited the unfortunate situations that arose during the hospitalization of your late wife to exemplify the many problems of administration and the lack of efficient care at the hospital.

As you may know, I am the chief sponsor of the Griffiths' Health Security Act, H.R. 22. This measure would provide complete coverage for practically every health care service at no direct charge to the patient. To control costs, hospitals would receive, after a process of negotiation, a predetermined annual budget under regulations, establishing the costs and services to be recognized in the budget. Financial incentives would be built into this program to encourage hospitals and individual physicians to keep people well rather than merely administering to their needs when they are ill. A uniform accounting system would be required, and the compensation of professional practitioners associated with hospitals would be tied to the hospital's budget. The budgetary guidelines and the financial incentives would serve to expedite the application of necessary treatment and eliminate unnecessary hospitalization.

Your comments and observations on the "system" of health care at University Hospital illustrate all too well the problems in the Nation's present system of health care delivery. In fact, the University Hospital is one of the better hospitals around, which emphasizes the need for reform in our current methods of delivering health care. My proposal would achieve this reform effectively, and assure all our citizens of receiving the health care they need at a price they can afford to pay.

Kind regards.

Sincerely,
Martha W. Griffiths
Member of Congress

I sent in reply the following:

Dear Mrs. Griffiths:

I genuinely appreciate your thoughtful letter of March 6 on the hospital/ medical situation.

Cost control in this field can be obtained only by bringing to the public view the real reasons for the excessive charges made which include:

1. Including in charges for bed time to patients expenditures having no legitimate bearing on costs of providing beds such as charges for student training and "research," a catchall for many unwarranted costs and a field of activity which itself warrants thorough investigation.

   If an organization which pays taxes to the state and operates as a profit-making facility could supply bed service in a semi-private room far superior to that afforded in wards at University Hospital, for $17 per day as against the $55 per day charged by this hospital, (now $71 per day) which is a *nonprofit* "state facility" and which *pays no taxes,* how can the hospital possibly account for the $38.00-a-day excess charge? They should certainly be required to clear this under the act you propose! The real and fundamental costs are the same for both. Any medical or laboratory service is a separate and extra charge in either case.

2. Laxity on the part of regents and hospital boards as to actual cost analysis. They apparently are overawed by the hospital/medical "elite" and serve simply as rubber stamps.

3. Greed and "salary and fees" status under which motivation the medical fraternity are out to get all they can with little regard to patient well-being. Dr. Knowles, now president of the Rockefeller Foundation was, I believe, conservative when he stated that 40 percent of doctors were "making a killing."

4. Lack of any controls by either state or federal agencies, failure of such agencies to get facts on costs and the fact that such agencies are largely manned and controlled by members of the medical monopoly.
5. Secret salaries paid by state facilities such as University Hospital serve to keep the public uninformed as to how their money is being spent and what they are getting for it— and also serves to send hospital charges to patients skyrocketing. $40,000 a year and up salaries should buy far better professional and management control!

I think your proposed objective of keeping people well rather than treat them after it is almost too late is sound, but keeping in mind Dr. Knowles's opinion that 40 percent of the doctors are more interested in the "fast buck" than in patient welfare, the prospect of attaining such a goal does not appear bright. As you wrote, University Hospital is one of the "better" facilities, yet the dollar standard of emulation is paramount here and the cost to and well being of the patient is definitely a secondary consideration.

A uniform accounting system will not correct the basic evils of the system unless it brings to light the *real cost element,* compares these costs with a standard in which every item is stated—and unless the *facts* are given to the public.

The fact that the medical monopoly restricts the output of doctors, thereby creating a shortage which overburdens the ethical and conscientious practitioner while creating a gold mine for the 40 percent not bothered with ethics should be acted on. Every university is a party to this "restraint of trade."

With best regards,
Rex Dye

I received a questionnaire from William S. Broomfield, M.C., and returned it with comment on the hospital medical problem. He responded as follows:

Dear Mr. Dye:
Thanks so much for your prompt reply to my questionnaire and for your additional comments on health care. I appreciate having your views on these matters which will be especially valuable to me when these issues are considered on the floor of the House of Representatives.

Your questionnaire will be tabulated along with those of the other residents of the 19th Congressional District. The results will be made known to the President and Congress. I will also be sending you a copy of the results so that you can compare your views with those of your neighbors.

As you know, there is legislation pending in Congress which would create a national health insurance program. These bills range from establishing a federally-financed and federally-administered health insurance program to encouraging or mandating the purchase of private health insurance plans meeting standards set by the federal government. If you have specific proposals on health care legislation, Mr. Dye, please let me know and I'll be happy to discuss them with the Chairman of the House Ways and Means Committee.

Best wishes,
William S. Broomfield, M.C.

My reply follows:

Dear Mr. Broomfield:

I am glad to get your letter of March 29, 1974, and appreciate your interest in the hospital-medical problem.

I do not feel that health care legislation is the answer (except in the case of "constitutional autonomy," a device permitting state hospitals associated with universities to maintain salary secrecy as to how they spend taxpayers' money and conceal other costs).

The solution I believe requires:

1. Investigation by competent efficiency engineers and cost analysts of *real costs* as compared to *charges to patients.*
2. Effective controls by state and federal agencies (now largely staffed at executive levels by members of A.M.A. and state medical societies highly unlikely to act in the public interest.
3. Full publicity so the public can know how they are being "taken."
4. Action by the Antitrust Division of the Department of Justice as to covert associative price-fixing by doctors, hospitals, drug suppliers, etc., and state and national lobbying by all groups in the health care industry.

I believe you are aware that in attempting to correct the abuses prevalent you will be opposed by one of the wealthiest and most highly organized political and economic forces in the nation, a group who were paid $17 billion in 1970 by the insurance industry alone according to Senator Kennedy in his book *In Critical Condition.* This group is in control of most state and city departments of health. They have state and national associations able to bring pressure to bear on members as in the case of Dr. John Knowles, now president of the Rockefeller Foundation, when the Massachusetts Medical Society censured him for publicly stating that 30 to 40 percent of doctors were "making a killing."

If you can get action on this, 5,000,000 people paying exorbitant Blue Cross premiums will owe you a vote of gratitude!

I have sent the accompanying and other data to Common Cause and
the Nader group. I feel that when the situation breaks it will make even
Watergate look like petty larceny by comparison.

Sincerely,
Rex Dye

You will note that I called Mr. Broomfield's attention to the political and economic force that public representatives would face in any
attempt to break this defacto monopoly. His reply follows:

Dear Mr. Dye:

Thank you for your recent letter in which you urge an investigation of
specific medical institutions such as university hospitals, implementation of
more effective controls in state and federal agencies as well as controls over
the influence of members of the health care industry.

I appreciate having your views on this urgent problem which will certainly be helpful to me in finding solutions to our health care problems.
Although I realize that you feel legislation would not solve these problems, I
thought you might be interested in the enclosed report on the Senate Labor
and Public Welfare Subcommittee on Health hearings dealing with the
revisions of health planning and regulations programs.

As you know, Senator Kennedy and Representative Mills have joined
to introduce a national health-insurance bill that, although more costly,
offers more liberal benefits than the administrative proposal. This measure will
include quality controls, insistence on health planning, compulsory coverage
of all Americans and operation through the Social Security System. While
not eliminating the health-insurance industry as in the original Kennedy
bill, the new bill gives it a restricted role as fiscal intermediary.

In the meantime, Mr. Dye, I will certainly study your allegations carefully and make your views known to the Secretary of Health, Education,
and Welfare. As soon as I receive his reply, I will let you know.

With all good wishes.

Sincerely,
William S. Broomfield

The report of the Senate Labor and Public Welfare Subcommittee
on Health hearings Mr. Broomfield enclosed with his letter had two
points of view, both of which overlooked the basic requirement for
any effective corrective action, namely the investigation of specific
health facilities by competent experts not subject to "influence" by the
hospital/medical forces, and full release to the press of findings. The
Watergate criminals and their undercover activity against the public

interest would never have been heard of without public disclosure by the nation's press.

Governor Philip W. Noel of Rhode Island felt that governors should have the option of designating local governments or regional bodies as area agencies for channeling of federal money within the state and also that some regulatory requirements be optional. This would certainly be highly desirable politically for the governor, but in view of the failure of state governments to control even the state hospital facilities operating under their aegis would be disastrous as far as the taxpaying public was concerned.

Russell B. Roth, president of the American Medical Association, whose chairman, John Kernodle, was indicted by a federal grand jury on charges of conspiracy and misapplying bank funds to the tune of nearly $1.8 million, opposed the Kennedy bill because of unprecedented federal involvement "in traditional responsibilities of state and local governments." He complained that the Kennedy bill would "stifle meaningful competition, innovation and development in the health care field." He apparently was not aware of the fact that no "meaningful competition" existed in this field.

No national health insurance bill can possibly solve the health care problem and protect the public against exorbitant costs, while hospitals and doctors are allowed to price their services far beyond real costs and so grossly inflate insurance actuarial experience on which any sound insurance must be based.

If a national health care insurance plan serves only as a collection agency to secure funds to pay the outlandish charges made for health care it will only create another bonanza for the money-hungry controllers of the health care industry.

Mr. Broomfield sent me a memo enclosing a reply he received from H.E.W. in response to data which I had supplied and which he had sent them.

The response from H.E.W. which follows is, again, a typical response from a bureaucracy to the taxpayers who pay the bureaucrats' salaries, passing the buck to Congress, with "concern and continuing efforts"!

Dear Mr. Broomfield:
Thank you for your letter of April 10 with which you forwarded a letter

from Mr. Rex Dye of Novi, Michigan, who delineates some hospital and medical practices of deep concern to him.

The federal government shares Mr. Dye's concern in these matters and is striving to develop a system of health care at a cost that will be within the reach of all Americans. We believe that one important step in this direction is the enactment of legislation to establish health maintenance organizations (HMOs) whose first critical objectives will be to more efficiently use medical manpower and to control soaring medical costs. Another initiative, the Professional Standards Review Organizations (PSROs), when established, will assure that health care paid for under Medicare, Medicaid and Maternal Child Health Programs is medically necessary, consistent with professionally recognized standards, and will encourage the use of less costly sites and modes of treatment, where medically appropriate. Also, there are a number of proposals before the Congress for the creation of a national health insurance system. One of these, the National Health Policy and Health Development Act of 1974, would give state health commissions broad regulatory powers including the power to regulate health institution rates.

We appreciate your interest in these vital health care issues and appreciate Mr. Dye's comments. You may be assured that we shall continue in our efforts to make full and equitable health care in this nation a reality.

Sincerely yours,
Cherry Y. Tsutsumida

How can any member of Congress serve his constituents when he or she has to deal with a bureaucracy? Any possible action is placed in the remote future under Parkinson's "Law of Delay"; the bureaucrat has tactfully sidestepped the issue and his salary continues!

Mr. Broomfield has my sympathy! I wrote him this letter:

Dear Mr. Broomfield:
Thanks for sending me the letter from H.E.W.

I'm sure you recognized it as a typical response from a bureaucracy on my question relating to the public interest—"The Federal Government Shares Concern," references to "HMO's," "PSRO's" action to give state health commissions "broad regulatory power" (these commissions are already under the control of the hospital/medical trust!) and ending with "you may be assured," etc.!

This reminds me of the 500-page "study"(!) of the "Technical Work on Health Care Costs" established by our Governor Milliken in 1971 titled, "Rising Medical Costs in Michigan." This group of 17 people spent hours of time, (the report was published in July 1973—two years later!) was of no value and accomplished nothing outside of getting the governor some publicity. One cost accountant and one efficiency engineer, fully empowered and turned loose in University Hospital could have produced a report which, *if publicized,* could have revolutionized health care in the state—at a fraction of the cost to them of this "study."

Sincerely,
Rex Dye

In July of 1971 I received a bulletin from Jack McDonald, congressional representative from the 19th Michigan district giving a summary of the results of a questionnaire he had mailed to 50,000 people in the district.

In response to question two of his questionnaire, "Are you in favor of a National Health Program for those who, regardless of age, cannot afford to pay medical expenses?" 55 percent of men, 59 percent of women, and 60 percent of the 18-21 age favored such a program. (The fact that the rate of increase in hospital/medical costs would place most of our population in the "cannot afford to pay" category was overlooked!)

I wrote Mr. McDonald:

Dear Mr. McDonald:

In your "Congressional Report" of July 1971, received at my home in Novi, your questionnaire response relative to a national health program "for those who, regardless of age, cannot afford to pay medical expenses" interested me.

I feel you should also ask (and get an answer) to the question of *why* they cannot pay medical/hospital expenses—and I feel very strongly that excessive charges by the medical/hospital combine are by far the largest single factor causing this condition.

I am enclosing data supporting this view as it applies to excessive hospital charges, which not only place a heavy burden on those who are uninsured, but also results in excessive premium rates to those insured under Blue Cross and similar programs.

If a national health program were to permit these continuing uncontrolled charges, no possible good could come to your constituents under such a plan.

Blue Cross, controlled by hospitals and doctors and other insuring programs, bases rates on inflated charges by hospitals and the medical fraternity. Over 5,000,000 people in Michigan are paying these excessive rates on Blue Cross alone!

If you will review the enclosed material as to bed charges I believe you'll find that an investigation of *real* costs and excessive billing is vital to any productive approach to the national health program.

Sincerely,
Rex Dye

The second paragraph of his letter in response indicates the failure of our legislators to recognize the fundamental problem involved.

Dear Mr. Dye:

Thank you so much for your letter of December 3, pertaining to a national health care program.

Hospital/medical expenses have risen due to the advances in science and in medical and health care techniques and, as other expenses, have risen due to the inflation throughout our economy. The cost of care has been driven to the point where provisions are excessive and persons of moderate or good income have been left economically drained or seriously in debt after a long illness. However, I firmly believe that once inflation has been stopped, the costs of all products, including the cost of medical care, will fall to a realistic level.

Briefly, under Medicredit the federal government pays the total premium for all those too poor to buy their own health insurance and offers a choice to those who can pay part—if not all—of their coverage between a graduated medical premium payment or a tax credit. In general, the less a person can afford to pay, the more the government helps out.

Medicredit and several other health care proposals are the subject of consideration before the House Ways and Means Committee. I shall work for the enactment of my bill or a compromise measure that will solve the financial dilemma of our health care industry. Your letter and the several enclosures on bed charges will be a great aid to me in this endeavor.

With kindest regards, I remain,

Sincerely yours,
Jack McDonald

I wrote Mr. McDonald again as follows:

Dear Mr. McDonald:

I was glad to get your letter of December 16th and to note your interest in the hospital/medical cost problem.

In the second paragraph of your letter you state that these expenses have risen due to advances in science, techniques and inflation generally . . . but I feel that you are overlooking the fundamental causes of the outrageous charges made . . . the facts (1) that hospital/medical insurance such as Blue Cross, largely under the control of hospital/medical groups has made it possible for the hospital/medical combine to extract exorbitant fees and charges from the public in a relatively "painless" manner; (2) that little or no state or federal controls have existed with regard to this monopolistic "industry"; (3) that hospital bed charges include excessive "costs" due to med-student training, "research" (a term which can cover a multitude of charges), excessive salaries of $40,000 a year or more on part-time jobs (note recent disclosure of salaries paid professors and administrators of medicine at Michigan State University—kept *secret* until disclosed by Bob Repas, a professor at the university! Taxpayers are apparently not supposed to know where their money goes!); (4) inefficient hospital management, overstaffing and excessive salaries.

The cost of hospital/medical care will not drop to realistic levels until *charges* made by this monopolistic group are based on realistic *costs* and until these *real* costs are disclosed to the public as the result of penetrating investigation by competent analysts not subject to influence from this powerful group.

Unless a real housecleaning occurs, Medicredit or similar plans would only serve as additional vehicles through which the hospital/medical combine could extract added millions of dollars from the public and would result in a substantially increased tax burden on the taxpayer who must finally pay the bill.

You have not had time to read and analyze the material I sent you and I feel sure that when you have been able to do so the imperative need for action that exists will become more clear.

It is my feeling that this whole subject will become a critical issue not only in Michigan and among your constituents but also nationally, and I believe it warrants the most thoughtful attention on the part of those we sent to Congress.

Sincerely,
Rex Dye

I sent Mr. McDonald some additional data bearing on the hospital/medical question to which he replied with the following letter.

Dear Mr. Dye:
Thank you so much for your letter of March 27. It was good to hear from you again.

As you may know, the House Ways and Means Committee is currently holding executive sessions on the various proposed health care plans; a clean bill, containing the best provisions of the plans, is expected to be reported out. I shall be certain to commend to my colleagues on that committee your letter and attachments regarding the investigation of real medical costs as opposed to artificial costs.

With kindest regards, I remain.

Sincerely yours,
Jack McDonald
Member of Congress

Mr. McDonald wrote again, enclosing a copy of a memorandum from the House Ways and Means Committee. His letter and the memorandum follow.

Dear Mr. Dye:

Enclosed is a copy of a memorandum I received today from the House Committee on Ways and Means regarding my recent inquiry in your behalf regarding the problems concerning health care costs. I believe that you will find the reply to be self-explanatory.

You may be sure that I will be following this legislation closely in the days ahead to see that some meaningful reforms are passed by the Congress.

I am glad to have had this opportunity to be of assistance and hope that you will continue to give me the benefit of your thinking on other issues in which you have interests.

With kindest regards, I remain,

Sincerely,
Jack McDonald
Member of Congress

Memorandum
To: Honorable Jack McDonald
From: Office of Minority Counsel
Re: Correspondence from Mr. Rex Dye (returned herewith)

Mr. Dye has submitted a number of newspaper articles, accompanied by commentary, illustrating problems with respect to health care costs today.

As you know, the Ways and Means Committee has held four and a half weeks of public hearings on pending legislation in the national health insurance area and is expected to resume deliberations in the next Congress. At that time, the Committee will be addressing itself to the problems indicated by Mr. Dye and you may wish to inform him that his helpful letter will be retained in our files and called to the attention of the Committee at the appropriate time.

You will see from the foregoing that the problem of getting corrective action through political channels is involved and time consuming! Material is referred to bureaus and committees, your material is helpful and will be retained in files—but what actually happens?

In 1971 I received a mailing from Senator Robert P. Griffin regarding a bill he had introduced in Congress to "authorize and encourage" railroads, bus lines, and air lines to reduce fares to senior citizens which he believed would cut such fares by as much as 50 percent. In his form letter he stated he did a lot of air traveling (at public expense?) and said he saw a lot of empty seats on air lines.

I wrote the senator:

Dear Senator:

Your letter of June 30, 1971, to my home in Novi regarding your Bill S-2055 interested me, but I frankly cannot regard this projected program as particularly vital . . . particularly in view of the fact that far more pressing problems exist which require action on the part of those in a position to act to solve them. Five million people in Michigan alone (including perhaps a majority of your constituents) are paying excessive health insurance rates to Blue Cross alone, as the result of excessive hospital/medical charges. Those without insurance are paying these excessive charges directly. Millions of dollars of excessive charges to Michigan voters are being channeled into the bank accounts of the hospital/medical combine annually—with no controls as to rates by either state or national bodies such as exist with other utilities and services to the public.

Keeping in mind that when these services are required by an individual, that individual and family are under serious emotional pressure. It is often a life or death situation and those who need these services are in no position to "shop" or consider the cost . . . they are at the mercy of the "supplier."

I believe that this problem will become a major issue soon and that effective controls are vital to a solution of the whole national health probem.

I am enclosing data which I believe you will find merits thoughtful study.

I am,

Sincerely,
Rex Dye

His response follows:

Dear Mr. Dye:
Thank you for your recent letter.

You will be interested to know the President's Economic Stabilization Council has frozen the Blue Cross/Blue Shield insurance rates.

In addition, the House Government Operations Committee is currently holding an investigation into this insurance plan.

I am grateful for the enclosures you have sent to me. Please be assured that I shall give them my close attention at first opportunity.

Your interest in writing is appreciated.

With best wishes and my kind regards, I am,

Sincerely,
Robert P. Griffin
U.S. Senator

I wrote him as follows:

Dear Senator:

I was glad to get your letter of December 9, 1971, and to note freezing of Blue Cross/Blue Shield rates.

This action does not, of course, imply any correction of the excessive charges being made by the hospital/medical combine. Blue Cross, Blue Shield, Medicare and other insurance programs as are now functioning only serve to enrich the hospital/medical people by establishing a method through which excessive charges can be extracted from the consumer "health market" in a relatively painless manner.

I am enclosing a preliminary chart [see Appendix 1] covering this operation and some additional news items bearing on the subject which I believe might serve as a starting point for intensive fact-gathering and investigation which could save the public nationally many millions of dollars annually—and result in vastly improved service to this viciously exploited market.

I am sincerely,
Rex Dye

To this letter he responded with the following letter. The political phrasing is obvious.

Dear Mr. Dye:

Many thanks for your most recent letter.

I share your concern about the need to improve the delivery of our health care services—and to devise better health insurance standards.

I've had a chance to skim the material you enclosed, and it is certainly interesting and absorbing. You may be assured that I shall give your suggestions most careful attention and consideration as Congress continues to consider this important topic.

With best wishes and my kind regards, I am,

Sincerely,
Robert P. Griffin
U.S. Senator

I mailed the senator additional data and in his response he still "shared my concern," "appreciated my interest," and gave me his "best wishes and kindest regards"!

Dear Mr. Dye:

Thanks for your recent letter and enclosures.

I share your concern regarding rising hospital costs. I am confident that the Senate will consider this matter, and you may be assured that I shall keep your views in mind.

Your interest in writing is appreciated.

With best wishes and my kind regards, I am,

> Sincerely,
> Robert P. Griffin
> U.S. Senator

What can your state or national senator or representative do to bring hospital/medical charges into line with charges for other products and services? If he or she takes a positive stand on this question how can they, as individuals, bring about on-the-spot hospital investigations as to efficiency and real costs? How can they curb such situations as pathologists taking up to $300,000 annually from laboratory charges? How can they bring adequate political power to bear to combat a $20 billion industry effectively? How can they get action out of powerful federal and state bureaucracies? Your legislator is virtually powerless to act effectively in your behalf as an individual when faced with such powerful political forces and buck-passing bureaucracy.

The extent of the American Medical Association's involvement in influencing legislation favorable to the medical industry is indicated by an Associated Press story appearing in the *Detroit Free Press* in October of 1974 in which Dr. W. J. Lewis, chairman of the American Medical Political Action Committee was reported as saying the committee would contribute approximately $600,000 to political campaigns this year.

The article further stated that organized medicine has contributed more than $400,000 to the campaigns of 42 House members, most of them supporters of the American Medical Association's health insurance proposal. It was stated that the 39 Republicans and 3 Democrats who shared this money voted for legislation favored by the American

Medical Association and against legislation the Health Security Action Council said would reform personal health care services.

It seems obvious that medical interests would not invest these substantial funds without expecting a substantial return—a return which must come out of the pockets of those requiring hospital and medical care.

9

Bureaucratic Aspects

Federal and state bureaucracies, operating under civil service, do most of the routine work of day-to-day governmental business. The word "routine" is significant as virtually every action in this sphere of government activity becomes a routine operation, much the same as a worker on a production line in an automobile factory, but with less control of output and a preponderance of "paperwork."

In my experience there seems to be little incentive to efficient operation under civil service. Job descriptions will include reference to authority over x number of people and as this degree of authority increases as to number of employees supervised, the rating and pay increase.

If a supervisor were so efficient and conscientious as to do the same amount of work with half the number of people, his authority would drop and so would his paycheck. If, on the other hand, he was able to do the same work with twice as many people, his rating would go up as would his pay—and the pay of his superior. It appears that civil service bureaucracies are automatically self-expanding and that efficiency is a secondary consideration.

Real authority appears to exist only at the higher levels with the result that matters requiring decision and action are passed up through channels to the top and then back down through channels to lower levels, departments, commissions, committees and other bureaus, with the result that no decisive action occurs and that the matter is effectively projected into the remote future. The issue has been successfully side-stepped and bureaucracy rolls on.

I wrote to the Detroit office of the Social Security Administration, enclosing material bearing on the hospital/medical problem. The letter follows:

91

Attention: Hospital Insurance and Medicare Section

Gentlemen:

The enclosed memo and data may be of interest with regard to costs of hospitalization to those coming under the federal Medicare program.

I do not know what action can be taken by your administration to investigate, bring to light, and curb practices which result in such price charges, but I believe any action that can be taken would certainly be in the public interest.

I am,

Sincerely,
Rex Dye

I received a reply from the regional office in Chicago which follows:

Dear Mr. Dye:

We are concerned about the care your wife received in the University Hospital, Ann Arbor, Michigan.

When we are advised that an accredited hospital may be furnishing poor care, we bring this to the attention of the Joint Commission on Accreditation of Hospitals. The Joint Commission conducts periodic surveys to assure that accredited hospitals are rendering high-quality care. Where the Commission removes accreditation, the Medicare program undertakes an independent investigation of the hospital to determine compliance with Medicare health and safety requirements and decides whether continued participation in the Medicare program should be permitted.

Your report about the care your wife received at University Hospital has been sent to the Joint Commission.

Sincerely yours,
Fred B. Wolf
Regional Representative
Health Insurance

I replied to this letter enclosing a copy of the letter from Mr. Zugich of University Hospital which stated my memo was "one of the most constructive which could be received by management."

Dear Mr. Wolf:

Your Ref: HI-5:8
Your letter 9/15/70

I am enclosing copy of letter from University Hospital, Ann Arbor, Michigan, received in response to the data sent you, subject reference number above.

This letter evidences the validity of my statements in memo sent you and indicates that efforts are underway to correct these highly undesirable conditions.

It is my feeling that the "reorganization" they state is underway should be under close observation by your Joint Commission to assure that proposed corrective action actually takes place and the real costs and charges are brought into a reasonable relationship.

Based on my experience, their charges are at least twice what they should be and I do not doubt that similar inequities exist in other hospitals greatly increasing the cost of Medicare.

Sincerely,
Rex Dye

I received the following letter in reply:

Dear Mr. Dye:

Thank you for your recent letter wherein you express concern over the high charge structure at the University Hospital. A point of clarification, however, should be made with respect to Medicare reimbursement.

Under the health insurance program for the aged, the amount paid to any provider of services e.g., hospital, extended care facility, or home health agency—for the covered services furnished to beneficiaries is the reasonable cost of such services, and not the charge of such services. This method is consistent with the prevailing practice of third party organizations. Although the Medicare program would be prohibited from forcing the provider to alter its charging practice, we can determine upon what basis we will reimburse.

Sincerely,
Fred B. Wolf
Regional Representative
Health Insurance

The data I had sent the Chicago office not only referred to the exorbitant price structure, but also, and even more important to the quality of service, needless bed time, invasion of privacy, and related malfunctionings. Nothing further developed from this correspondence.

I sent the following letter to the Secretary of Health, Education and Welfare, with a rather complete file of data such as has been given in previous chapters of this book.

Dear Mr. Richardson:
I am submitting herewith a file on hospital/doctor costs which may be of

interest in connection with your development of controls on costs of such services.

This field appears to me to be highly monopolistic in character with charges and fees having little relation to real costs, with little, if any, competitive price controls and with tacit understandings between hospitals, doctors and insurors as to getting every dollar they can from the public in the form of hospital charges, medical fees and insurance premiums.

I am sincerely,
Rex Dye

This was "bucked" down to a "lower channel of authority" as follows:

Dear Mr. Dye:
The Secretary has asked me to reply to your letter about rising medical costs.

We are giving your letter attention and will be in touch with you again as soon as possible.

Sincerely yours,
Robert M. Ball
Commissioner of Social Security

I later received the following communication:

Dear Mr. Dye:
This is in further response to your letter to Secretary Richardson about rising medical costs.

We found the file on hospital and doctor costs that you enclosed with your letter to be of much interest, and we thank you for giving us the benefit of your views and experiences on this important subject. We will certainly take them into full consideration in our continuing studies of ways to provide health care services as economically as possible, while maintaining or improving the quality of such service.

We agree that there is a pressing need to slow down the rate of increase in the costs of health care. I'm sure you realize that this requires cooperate efforts on the part of those who provide the health services, as well as those who provide the financing for such services—including the general public, the Government (Federal, State, and local) and private insurance.

The Department of Health, Education, and Welfare is making special efforts to attack the problem through the Medicare program, as well as on the broader front of all Department programs. We recognize the problems inherent in the Medicare cost reimbursement formula, and we are attempting to overcome them. We have instituted an incentive reimbursement experimentation program which is designed to test, under controlled conditions, the various alternatives to the cost reimbursement method. Incentive payments will be made to hospitals and other providers of services to induce them to introduce cost control measures which show promise of controlling the rapid escalation of medical care costs. As this is a relatively new program, none of the experiments have been completed and no results are available as yet.

Thanks again for your report on the matter, Mr. Dye. We appreciate very much your passing it on to us.

Sincerely yours,
Robert M. Ball
Commissioner of Social Security

I later sent Mr. Ball additional information with this letter of transmission:

Gentlemen:
With further regard to your letter of January, 1972, I am enclosing additional data bearing on the file on hospital/medical costs which I sent to Mr. Richardson in December of 1971.

The chart I am enclosing [see Appendix 1] represents an initial approach to an analysis of the hospital/medical combine on which further supporting data can be based and organized for effective corrective action.

The file I previously sent you bears out the outline developed in this chart as do the additional news items enclosed. If newspapers were checked nationally and items classified with relation to enclosed chart data, a very conclusive case would be had in a short time.

I am sincerely,
Rex Dye

The reply follows:

Dear Mr. Dye:
This is in response to your latest letter and previous correspondence concerning medical costs.

Thank you for the additional material you sent us regarding hospital/medical costs. We appreciate your interest in this important matter and we will give it full consideration in our continuing effort to provide quality care as economically as possible.

Sincerely yours,
Robert M. Ball
Commissioner of Social Security

To my knowledge no positive action was taken—and hospital

charges kept skyrocketing, the daily charge for a ward bed at University Hospital having soared to $71 per day in 1972 from $50 per day in 1970.

I sent data on hospital prices to the Price Commission, executive office of the president, at Washington, D.C., with the following letter:

Dear Mr. Grayson:
I am enclosing data bearing on excessive prices being charged on hospital/medical services which may have a bearing.

You may note from the chart showing price rises on hospital services from U.S. Department of Labor statistics that the rate of increase has been more than double that of "all items" category (utilities, food prices, wages of rank and file personnel, heating, office equipment, etc.), the outrageous price increases do not reflect *actual* costs but rather the greed and mismanagement of an economic activity extracting hundreds of millions of dollars from the public annually through excessive billings having little relation to fair pricing based on costs under efficient management.

The accompanying preliminary analysis chart of the hospital/medical combine indicates an approach to control of this monopolistic activity.

A file of newspaper clippings from papers nationally, keyed to various aspects of this chart, would develop quite conclusive evidence on this subject in a relatively short time, I believe.

The few clippings enclosed point strongly to the condition existing.
I am,

Sincerely,
Rex Dye

Here again the problem was "bucked" down to a lower level for attention. You will note that the "Health Services Committee," appointed by the president to advise the "Cost of Living Council" and the "Pay Board" and that my "information" and "interest" was appreciated."

Dear Mr. Dye:
Chairman Grayson asked that I reply to your recent letter.

We have recognized the inflation that has been plaguing the health area as well as the entire economy. Because the health industry has been one of the leaders in the increase in cost of living in recent years, special regulations were developed for them, Sections 300.18 and 300.19 of our Economic Stabilization Regulations.

We have had the advice of the Health Services Industry Committee, a

Presidentially appointed Committee to advise the Cost of Living Council, the Price Commission, and the Pay Board.

We are confident that our efforts in this area are going to be successful in lowering the increase in the cost of health services. The preliminary statistics are favorable but it's too soon to declare the battle won.

We've appreciated the information that you've given us, and we also appreciate your interest in the fight to stop the inflation.

Sincerely,
Louis P. Neeb
Executive Secretary

I sent some further data later to Mr. Neeb, whose acknowledgment follows:

Dear Mr. Dye:
Thank you for your note of June 24 with the additional information. We are always interested in the views of the public in the area of Economic Stabilization. We noted carefully the points that you have made in your letter to Mr. McCann [see Chapter 4] along with the markings on the various other enclosures.

I trust that you have been reading the current consumer price indexes and have noted that there has been a considerable decrease in the health care component of that index from the period prior to the Economic Stabilization Program.

Sincerely,
Louis P. Neeb
Executive Secretary

In response to additional data sent Mr. Neeb he responded as follows:

Dear Mr. Dye:
Thank you for the information that you sent to us.

I think you are addressing this data to the wrong agency. The Price Commission has a general mandate to control prices. Our mandate does not extend to looking into the whys and wherefores of medical or health practice. There are a number of congressional committees and other departments of the Federal Government involved in this area and, as you are aware, there were a number of national health proposals before the last Congress. Of course, they'll have to be renewed when the new Congress goes into session towards the end of January.

The Consumer Price Index indicates that we're having considerable success in the health area. The overall health services portion has been reduced to almost a third of what it was prior to the institution of the Economic Stabilization Program. This would indicate to us that, from an overall standpoint, we have obtained our goal.

Some of the issues you raised and the enclosures, with your letter, concern such things as method and approach to practice. We are not authorized nor are we able to judge one doctor's charging pattern against another, as long as it does not violate our guidelines.

As always, we do appreciate your interest.

Sincerely,
Louis P. Neeb
Executive Secretary

I replied:

Dear Mr. Neeb:

I genuinely appreciate your letter of 11/7/72 and thank you for writing me so fully.

I realize that some of the data I sent did not relate solely to prices but I believe that the three specific cases instanced by the enclosures herewith warrant consideration by your commission.

(A) An increase in bed charges of 42 percent from 1970 to 1972. In view of the fact that all basic *real* costs are included in the "all items" category of U.S. Department of Labor statistics, the 200 percent increase of hospital charge as against a 40 percent increase in "all items" seems to me totally unwarranted. When you add the University Hospital increase since 1970 of 42 percent far beyond any *normal* inflation, it seems to me that investigation is called for.

(B) When one doctor charges $15 for a hearing test and another charges $5 for the *same* test (but much more thorough!) it seems to me that, aside from the manner in which the test was given and even if both were equally thorough, the price difference warrants investigation as the $15 figure (twice that allowed under Medicare) is highly inflated and billing of this order can only be strongly inflationary.

(C) When hospitals provide the "plush" service noted in this item, including parlor with bar, remote control T.V., bedroom with rolltop desk, special direct-dial telephone, sofa bed for use of family for *only* $102 per day as compared with *ward bed,* NO PARLOR, NO BEDROOM, NO BAR, NO T.V., NO TELEPHONE, NO DESK, NO SOFA BED, NO SPECIAL SERVICE, AND ABOUT 1/10 THE SPACE or less for $55 per day it seems to me you have a price situation in which ward patients are grossly overcharged and which should be given attention by your commission as I believe you will find this condition general, resulting more contributing to the highly inflationary charges which have characterized hospital billing.

Regards,
Rex Dye

No further communication has been received, in fact I do not know whether or not this operation in the president's office still exists.

10

Other Economic Aspects

Excessive health care costs hit not only the pocketbooks and bank accounts of hospital patients and those paying insurance premiums for health care coverage as the result of insurance rates based on inflated hospital "costs" which include such hidden charges as "research" and training of medical students, but also are reflected in the selling prices of all consumer goods where the employer pays for health insurance coverage on behalf of employees.

For example, when Mr. McKenna of the Ford Motor Company said Ford premiums for such insurance increased from $41.69 for each employee per month in 1970 to $66.09 in 1972 (and further increases have occurred in 1973 and 1974), he was stating that the cost of producing an automobile had increased. When the cost of processing the needed records, overhead, space required and legitimate profit are added to this basic figure it will be seen that the price to the consumer must rise substantially and that it is the consumer who finally pays. Other automobile manufacturers, and all other employers acting as collecting agencies for the hospital/medical combine, face parallel cost problems and must pass these costs on to the public in pricing their products. Increases of two to three times labor costs on the part of industry are necessary to cover overhead and produce a legitimate profit, and, as any fringe benefits such as hospital insurance are a direct labor cost, consumers must pay from two to three times the amount garnered by health insurors in premiums. The general effect of this exploitation of the health market can only be grossly inflationary.

I wrote Mr. Iacocca of the Ford Motor Company, who was chairman of the United Foundation Capital Fund Division Campaign in 1972, enclosing data on the hospital/medical problem.

Dear Mr. Iacocca:
I read with interest the news story regarding hospital financing and while I am in hearty accord with any action to relieve human suffering and its attendant costs, I believe there are some aspects of this overall situation that should be given thoughtful attention before commitments are made.

The enclosed material outlines some of the existing conditions which should be corrected.

You will, I believe, find this material worth thoughtful reading.

I am,

Sincerely,
Rex Dye

I received the following response:

Dear Mr. Dye:
Mr. Iacocca very much appreciated your letter and enclosed materials about hospital care.

Your deep personal concern about the problem, your obvious willingness to research the facts and your logical and clear presentation of them are a great, great credit to you personally. Hopefully they will help us toward better solutions to our health care problems. In this connection, Mr. Iacocca has asked me to forward your enclosures to the United Foundation's hospital committee. (As you are no doubt aware, however, the metropolitan UF does not extend to the University of Michigan Hospital in Ann Arbor).

Of course, Mr. Iacocca's concern currently is with raising funds for the United Foundation's Capital Fund Division, which supports construction and new equipment not only for hospitals but for 35 UF agencies, including the Salvation Army, the Cancer Foundation and Goodwill Industries, etc.

Thank you again for writing.

Sincerely,
Mott B. Heath

I wrote Mr. Heath as follows:

Dear Mr. Heath:
I was glad to get your letter of May 1, 1972, and to hear of Mr. Iacocca's interest in the enclosures.

I realize the Metro U.F. does not extend to University Hospital, but, as conditions there seem general among hospitals, I feel that action at a high enough level may bring a general corrective action.

University Hospital is a state facility paying no taxes and should set a standard which could be a model for other hospitals as to patient care, overall efficiency and realistic charges to patients for service rendered. In my experience, this is not the case.

I have some experience with control methods. Many years ago, I was employed as assistant to the superintendent of construction on a housing project of the Ford interest out Michigan Avenue, a Mr. Walstrum, if my memory serves me.

We were "losing" hardware on homes under construction. I developed a wall chart with model numbers at one side and parts used across the top. When a man came in for a given lock, etc., we gave him the material and put his badge number and date in the square where house number and part used intersected. The losses stopped.

During World War II, I was called to the federal building and asked to establish a reporting system at Fort Wayne Ordnance Depot. The operation was a mess. I set up a Control Staff, devised a cost control system based on man-hours applied to various work units such as line items, tons, etc. This started at foreman level, was consolidated at each higher level, ending up with a consolidated depot report by divisions giving week's performance against prior week. Depot output more than doubled with a man-hour savings in excess of $500,000 per month. [See Appendix 2; 3.]

The lack of organization and operating control I observed in this hospital was worse than the Ordnance Department! When viewed in the light of needless human suffering, excessive bed time at exorbitant charges and excessive insurance rates this condition is alarming.

The *Detroit Free Press* ran an item on $40,000-a-year-and-up salaries paid to professors and administrators of medicine at Michigan State University. I wrote University Hospital for data on salaries paid. No information has been forthcoming. A similar request to Governor Milliken has brought no response. As this is a state facility paying no taxes and therefore heavily subsidized by those who do, I feel such information should be readily available to any taxpayer.

No state facility should have any secret payrolls nor should taxpayers be expected to give these people a blank check.

The cost to industry annually in terms of lost mass consumer buying power due to excessive hospital/medical insurance rates *alone* must run into hundreds of millions of dollars annually. Blue Cross alone has 5,000,000 insured just in Michigan. And apparently excessive hospital billing is paid by insurors without question—they simpy boost rates to cover the charges!

It seems to me that state and national action to bring this situation under control has been very lax. If a similar situation existed in the auto industry the powers would be on your back like a ton of bricks!

I am sincerely,
Rex Dye

An inquiry to the greater Detroit Chamber of Commerce as to attaining information on salaries paid at University Hospital resulted in the following reply:

Thanks, Mr. Dye . . .
. . . for your letter of recent date. I am unable, from many sources available to me, to obtain the information you wish. I also talked to Lou Marr about the problem, and he says that as far as he knows the figures are still unavailable. I agree with you that the figures certainly should be available to the public since that is the source from which they received the funds.
Sorry I can't help further.

Cordially,
John R. Steiner, CCE
Manager
Research and Information

When state facilities are able to spend the taxpayers' money in secrecy, how can officials in government expect the public to have confidence that their money is not being misspent?

I wrote the Detroit Chamber of Commerce the following:

Jack,
I'm wondering if Governor Milliken's office would refuse the information re payrolls to the Chamber of Commerce if you were to write asking for this information. It doesn't seem right that this information should be withheld unless there is something to hide—and it raises a question in my mind as to what other expenditures of taxpayers' money are being covered up.
This is a flagrant action by a bureaucratic group to conceal from the public where taxpayers' money goes and shows a contemptuous disregard of that public of which you and I are a part.
Although the payroll is provided by us they apparently feel that they are a privileged group not accountable to those who foot their bills! If such figures are not made available on cost of state government operation any research is nullified before it starts.

Rex Dye

When information on spending by a state hospital facility funded by the public is not available to a Chamber of Commerce representing a state's business interests and employers, what chance has the general public to learn how and where their money goes!

The $20 billion a year, high profit health industry has a fearful impact on the national economy and results in a concentration of uncontrolled economic and political power that is frightening.

The health industry has plenty of money for high salaries, widespread advertising and "public relations" activity, lobby, political support and pressure as well as other "influence" action.

When to the direct charges to patients and heatlh providers, such as hospitals, are added the indirect charges on consumer goods resulting from inflated hospital and medical insurance premiums paid by employers, the cost to the general public becomes staggering!

It is becoming a serious question whether the national economy can continue to pay the tribute being exacted by this monopolistic elite. The time seems to be drawing nearer when only the privileged few can afford proper health care.

11

Racket Aspects

When the incentive of honest, ethical service at a fair market price based on legitimate costs to secure a fair and reasonable profit is replaced by the incentive to get the dollar, without regard to honesty, ethics, or morality, any business or professional activity degenerates to the level of racketeering. When the dollar motivation and standards of emulation supersede the desire for recognition based on accomplishment in the arts, science, industry, medicine and worthy craftsmanship; when the standing of a man is based on his dollar wealth instead of the quality of his contribution to the well-being of his fellow men; then racketeering develops. The deciding factor in any action becomes not the answer to "Is it the right thing to do morally and ethically?" but the affirmative answer to, "Can I or we get away with it?"

Had Mr. Connors (former director of University Hospital at Ann Arbor) answered this question of double billing negatively on the first question he would not have been forced to resign from this lucrative position. But he thought he could "get away with it." He did for three years, but an unexplained audit brought his dereliction to light.

Had Mr. John Kernodle, board chairman of the American Medical Association, answered this first question negatively when dealing with bank funds he would not have been indicted by a federal grand jury on charges of conspiracy and misapplying bank funds.

When Dr. Sidney Wolfe, a Ralph Nader associate, told the Commission on Medical Malpractice that at least 10,000 Americans die annually as a result of 2,000,000 unnecessary surgical operations, he was giving shocking evidence of the extent to which dollar motivation has replaced ethical service motivation. War is not as costly to the nation in human lives! Nor the murders committed by hardened criminals!

Had Dr. Jesse Ketchum, before establishing his ten-year-record of malpractice, considered the question of morality and ethics and decided to be honest and true to his oath as a doctor, he would not have been ordered to stop practicing in Michigan nor have been convicted for leaving a needle in the throat of a thirteen-year-old patient to be discovered two years later by another doctor. Yet his peers in the medical profession apparently took no action to prevent this doctor from practicing. Perhaps they did not want to "rock the boat."

Consumer advocate Ralph Nader, speaking at the 45th Annual Clinical Assembly of Osteopathic Specialists said the American medical and hospital patient may be the most frustrated and intimidated in the world, discouraged from asking doctors or hospitals about the care received. Intimidation is, of course, an obvious weapon of the racketeer—yet doctors themselves are intimidated by the fear of censure from their associations and societies if they speak out against abuses existing in their profession!

Billing by hospitals for services not rendered is certainly a form of larceny, yet an insurance company claims a supervisor was reported in the *Detroit Free Press* as saying that about ten percent of the claims paid were for services not rendered. Ruth Winter, in her book *How to Reduce Your Medical Bills,* states that errors or bill-padding by hospitals can cost you money and that one reason for the variation in hospital charges was evidently how much the hospital was willing to pad your bill. She also goes into the question of outlandish drug profiteering thoroughly.

The victims of the hospital/medical combine, faced with life or death situations and the desperate fear of the unknown, constitute an ideal market for exploitation by those who take advantage of their ignorance of medical problems and their desperation. There is no competition among providers of health care nor is there a free choice by the consumer; he is kept in ignorance and cannot judge the quality or pricing of the services available; he cannot make an informed choice as would be the case in other purchases; he is at the mercy of the monopoly.

He pays whatever is asked, "or else." If he cannot come up with the money, many hospitals will not admit him. And if the bill runs beyond his ability to pay he may be hounded into bankruptcy. Senator Kennedy's book *In Critical Condition* gives case records of this.

Hospitals do not hesitate to include and conceal in their billing charges that have no relation to the welfare of the patient, such as student training and "research." Why should a patient in a hospital be forced to contribute cash to the education of students in medicine or nursing? In so doing the patient is forced to pay for a service to the student which has no bearing whatever on the medical problem of that patient—and the patient becomes a guinea pig for the students' training. The patient should be paid for providing this training experience to the student! If the case is "interesting," even though terminal, the patient may be forced to endure a longer stay in the hospital so that students can watch its development. Of course, the patient would be billed for his additional time in the hospital.

Local, state and national health commissions, departments of public health and similar agencies are largely headed by medical men, subject to powerful influence on the part of local, state and national medical associations and societies. The hospital/medical combine virtually exercises control over the agencies who are supposed to control their activities. The effectiveness of this political control by the hospital/medical forces is evidenced by the fact that little or no action has been taken by these political representatives of the health industry to correct the flagrant abuses that exist or to in any way check the consciencelessness exploitation of the helpless health market.

Local, state and national agencies dealing with health and hospital control are highly unlikely to take any action in the public interest which might offend or reflect on those powerful interests in control of the medical profession. Few state or national legislators will have the courage to challenge this affluent political force with its network of political connections, its publicity men, its lobbyists and its abundance of funds.

Common Cause reported that the American Medical Association had $1.8 million in lobby funds according to a news item in the *Detroit Free Press,* July 11, 1974. When to this figure, the funds of related medical and hospital associations and those of individual hospitals are added, the political impact is obvious.

Medical men holding political positions such as health commissioners, heads of departments of health and similar political agencies are faced with the problem of conflict of interest as soon as they accept their appointments; the public interest versus the interests of the hospital/medical groups. The present state of health care in the United States seems to be ample evidence of the interest they have chosen to support.

How these individuals got their appointments, who appointed them, who influenced their appointment and what political and financial pressures were involved would be highly interesting and perhaps bring to light one of the major causes of the critical condition of health care in the United States today.

The selection of "public" members of the board at Blue Cross in Michigan from lists prepared by hospitals indicates the concern actually held for the public interest!

The fact that the conditions existing in the health care field are the result of the greed, coercion, exploitation and lust for power and prestige of a minority engaged in the health care field is, in itself, alarming. The fact that the majority apparently accepts this autocratic control and keeps silent is even more alarming.

12

Corrective Action

If hospital and medical associations are unable, unwilling or power-less to bring about effective action to correct the conditions which have created the crisis in health care, public pressure is likely to result in some form of socialized medicine—and then heaven help us! All that can be expected from governmental bureaucracies is in-creased costs, confusion and political mismanagement.

State and federal committees will produce more and more costly, verbose and time-consuming reports as the result of politically slanted hearings and "investigations" at taxpayer expense. State and federal bureaucrats will come under the domination of the hospital/medical monopoly as will the rank and file of doctors and hospital personnel.

Corrective action should come from within the medical profession itself; from the 60 to 70 percent of the doctors who are not out to "make a killing" and who are ethical and honorable in their practice. The existing abuses in the health care field place these members of the profession under unjustified suspicion and they should act to remove this reflection on their integrity. They should become active in the functioning of their medical societies and associations and clean house where housecleaning is necessary. The time is past when they can iso-late themselves from the growing problems of health care delivery even though they have established a sound practice in their own communities. For the young doctor, a recent graduate from medical school, the question is far more relevant and critical because his whole professional future is at stake. His experience as an intern should have made him aware of many of the evils of hospital operation. His con-tact with the professors of medicine during his college years should have given him an insight into the outdated and inflexible academic viewpoints on health care, medical training and objectives. He must decide whether his motivation in practice is to be that of the "fast buck artist" or honest service to humanity. And he must decide whether he is to accept conditions as they now exist in health care or to act to correct these conditions.

Rightminded hospital/medical practitioners cannot bring about the critically needed corrective action without public support. Every person paying excessive health insurance premiums (and this includes everyone who is insured), everyone who has paid excessive hospital bed and laboratory billings and everyone interested in competent, available health care at reasonable cost should give this support gladly!

Keeping in mind that hospital/medical personnel are subject to intense pressure and coercion from the multi-billion-dollar "health industry," you will realize that your individual efforts to secure corrective action can have little effect alone but you will realize, too, that when you affiliate with such consumer-oriented organizations working in the public interest as Common Cause, the Nader organization and consumer interest groups in your area, your voice can be heard.

I believe that everyone interested in better health care at far lower costs should support such groups and stipulate that correction of evils existing in the health care field be given top priority in group action.

Politicians want your vote. They want to stay in office. They will send you letters "appreciating your interest in this serious problem," but nothing will happen as the result of your appeal *as an individual*. But when that politician is confronted with demands made by an organization of many members, the vote count is a different story. It may be enough to outweigh the pressures of hospital/medical and insurance lobbies, advertising and other forms of "influence."

The cost of annual membership in these organizations will probably be less than you are now losing every month in excessive health insurance premiums, grossly inflated medical fees, and higher prices on consumer goods due to the inclusion of health insurance in labor production costs.

Write your local newspaper when you have been dealt with unfairly by a member of the hospital/medical group who is out to "make a killing." "Action Line" in the *Detroit Free Press* has run many such letters and obtained refunds of overcharges and other corrective action.

"Letters to the Editor" in this same paper have placed many examples of exorbitant charges and related evils in health care before the public. In writing to your newspaper, state your case clearly with dates, costs, overcharges, instances of poor service, insurance troubles and other examples of poor and costly hospital/medical care. Editors are aware of the critical state health care has reached in America and will respond to reader concern on this serious problem.

Write your local and national legislators, medical societies and health commissioners—but don't expect much in the way of immediate results. You are competing with one of the most powerful combines in the nation for their attention and interest and only when a tidal wave of public interest and indignation becomes evident can you expect action.

Action that should be taken includes:

(1) Elimination of secrecy on the part of state hospitals as to salaries and financial operations. In Michigan the taxpayer is prevented from knowing where his money goes by the device of "constitutional autonomy," which, in practice, constitutes a license to state universities and allied hospitals to spend taxpayers' money as they see fit, with no accountability to the taxpayer who pays the substantial salaries of the "educators," medical doctors and administrators involved. This secret spending privilege opens the door to many abuses.

(2) Every state hospital should be subject to annual audits and periodic checking of expenditures by the state auditor general. Such audits would prevent occurrences as the double billing for travel by Edward J. Connors, former director of University Hospital—over a period of several years—and might reveal and prevent other and possibly more serious misuse of taxpayers' money.

(3) The term "research" can cover a wide range of wasted funds charged to health care. A thorough investigation of "research" activities would, I believe, be revealing. The results of such an investigation should be made public. Answers to such questions as:

(a) What are the *specific* objectives of all specific medical research groups?

(b) How much time does each member of such a group actually spend on the job?

(c) What are the salaries paid?

(d) What is the total annual cost?

(e) What specific results are obtained? Progress reports should be made public.

(f) What is the cost factor of "research" applied to bed charges at such an institution as University Hospital, Ann Arbor, Michigan. All research projects should be subject to audit by state auditor general where tax-payer funds are involved.

(4) Student training at hospitals such as the University Hospital at Ann Arbor, Michigan, a state facility, should be thoroughly investigated. This training is directly a service to the student, not to the patient, yet the patient or his insuror foots the bill. What is the cost factor of student training applied to bed charges at hospitals?

(5) The insurance question should be investigated and the findings made public. Such an investigation should include: A study of the validity of actuarial experience involved with particular regard to charges by hospitals for "research," student training, "freedom funds" used by trustees or others, excessive bed charges as compared with convalescent homes giving far superior service such as the instance cited in chapter 2 of this book, "investments" of excess funds or "profits" by nonprofit organizations such as cited in chapter 3, and payments for services not rendered as cited in chapter 11.

(6) Patients should have the right to a detailed explanation of their hospital bills regardless of whether or not an insurance company is paying the bill and should have access to the hospital's records. Electrostats of hospital or doctors' case records could be made available to the patient at very little cost.

(7) No one not directly involved in the patient's care should be allowed in his hospital room or ward space without patient's permission. Students, visitors being given a grand tour of the hospital by hospital management, should be definitely excluded. The patient is not in the hospital to assist as a guinea pig in student training nor to be an exhibit on display to impress visiting doctors or other "dignitaries" with the hospital's facilities.

Action as outlined above is unlikely to be taken voluntarily by the hospital/medical combine. An aroused and well-publicized public opinion combined with action by effective consumer/taxpayer interest groups will be necessary to bring the existing crisis in health care under control.

But there are some actions you can take that will help secure this public opinion and impress it upon the attention of those in a position to act in your area.

If you or a family member are in a hospital and the call button signal is not answered in a reasonable time, say three minutes, tell your doctor, your relatives, your visiting friends. At the outrageous price you are being charged for a bed and due to the fact that you *are* in bed you should not submit to the needless suffering such callous disregard of your condition can cause. If student doctors or individuals of "teams" start asking the same questions regarding your condition, tell your doctor, relatives and friends and ask that this persecution be stopped. If you are subjected to any other infringement of your rights as a human being again tell your doctor, relatives and friends—they can do something about it.

If you make an appointment with a doctor for a specific time and are kept waiting over fifteen minutes with no explanation of the delay, tell the receptionist that you are sorry the doctor could not keep the appointment and leave. If the doctor has made so many appointments that he has a waiting room so full of patients that he cannot handle them properly you can be reasonably sure that his mind and attention will be on those in the waiting room rather than on your problems. You will probably be better off to seek another doctor, but before making an appointment ask if he keeps his appointments. If patients did this many waiting rooms would be empty and many needless follow-up office calls would be unnecessary as doctors would spend enough time with a patient to give a valid diagnosis and treatment, something not to be expected in a production-line operation where the objective is getting as many patients as possible through the mill and getting the highest dollar volume of "sales."

The foregoing applies to the 30 to 40 percent of doctors out to "make a killing," motivated by dollar income rather than service to the patient. In my experience you will find more of this type of operator among "specialists" than in those engaged in general or family practice. The 60 to 70 percent of doctors who are service oriented and motivated, should support patients' action to end the money hungry exploitation of the sick by unscrupulous hospital/medical groups motivated by desires for money and "status" in their practice, rather than to contribute to the alleviation of human suffering.

I believe that effective corrective action to bring the health care crisis under control can only be brought about through the cooperation of those rightminded members of the medical profession and an aroused public supported by strong public interest groups and the press. Governmental action will follow at state and national levels when this occurs.

Appendices

APPENDIX 1

PRELIMINARY CHART OF HOSPITAL/MEDICAL COMBINE — *for further investigation & analysis*

NATIONAL CONTROLS — — — STATE CONTROLS

Virtually nonexistent. Now beginning to receive attention due to critical increases in medical fees, hospital charges and prices of drugs.

Ineffective due to lack of thorough investigation of real costs — staffing of some agencies by medically oriented personnel — influence of hospital/medical fraternity on such agencies.

NATIONAL, STATE AND LOCAL MEDICAL AND HOSPITAL ASSOCIATIONS AND SOCIETIES

"PUBLIC RELATIONS" — Lobbying — Influence over hospital/medical legislation and national and state controls over hospital/medical activities.

MEDICAL COLLEGES

Excessive salaries to medical professors and administrators of medicine. Restricted "output" of M.D.'s due to such factors as archaic medical, anatomical and drug terminology and nomenclature; adherence to arbitrary and inefficient procedures; maintenance of rarified professional atmosphere similar to cult or secret society from which patients and public are excluded.

STUDENT AND INTERN EDUCATION AND TRAINING

(Sick patients and insured people should not be forced to donate to these activities)

HOSPITALS

Basic Function — Efficient, considerate care of patients at lowest possible cost.

EXCESSIVE CHARGES TO PATIENTS DUE TO: Excessive payrolls — Percentage deals with pathologists on laboratory work — Lack of efficient personnel and management controls — Charging patients for costs and expenses not properly an obligation of the patient such as student training, "research," etc., etc.

DEHUMANIZING OF SERVICE TO PATIENT: Patient regarded by hospital personnel as case number rather than as a human being — Failure and delay in responding to bed call button — Subjecting patient to unnecessary duplication of care questioning by interns — Disregard of patient comfort, peace of mind or well-being — Delay in arriving at diagnosis. CONTROL BY MEDICAL MINDS RATHER THAN EFFICIENCY ORIENTED MANAGEMENT.

"RESEARCH"

Cost elements in this category should be closely examined by competent cost analysts and investigators

HOSPITAL/MEDICAL—DRUGS, EQUIPMENT, SUPPLIES (PRODUCERS AND DISTRIBUTORS OF)

- Brand names at excessive prices as opposed to generic nomenclature
- High cost promotion, "detailing," etc.
- Excessive prices for instruments, lab equipment and apparatus, inefficient purchasing by hospital/medical groups
- Suppliers know this market is the "big money" and price wares accordingly

DOCTORS

- Excessive charges on Medicare-Medicaid-Blue Cross and other insurance programs.
- Lack of proper diagnosis and treatment.
- "Production Line" methods of handling patients on office calls to get greatest possible dollar volume in shortest possible time.

INSURORS

Premium rates based on uncontrolled and largely unquestioned charges by hospital/medical combination. Operation largely controlled by hospital/medical people. Insurors such as Blue Cross have opportunity served as vehicles enabling the hospital/medical combine to extract excessive charges from the huge "health" market in a relatively inconspicuous and "painless" manner.

Premium rates based on uncontrolled and largely unquestioned charges by hospital/medical combination.

"Public" representatives to Blue Cross Board selected in Michigan from list submitted by hospitals.

PREMIUM DOLLARS

5,000,000 BLUE CROSS INSURED IN MICHIGAN ALONE (PLUS OTHER INSURORS)

INSURED — NOT REQUIRING HOSPITAL/MEDICAL CARE

A CAPTIVE MARKET FOR HOSPITAL/MEDICAL INDUSTRY • LARGELY NON-COMPETITIVE AND LARGELY UNDER MONOPOLISTIC CONTROL. MARKET IS KEPT IN IGNORANCE OF "PRODUCT" THEY PAY FOR — CANNOT "SHOP" IN A COMPETITIVE MARKET AS WITH OTHER PRODUCTS.

Sick people are in no physical or mental state to bargain. They seek help without regard to cost and are extremely vulnerable marketwise. Obscure medical terminology, drug nomenclature and incomprehensible prescriptions combine with fear, uncertainty and emotional pressure to create an atmosphere of bewilderment and often desperation. Such a market should be protected from exploitation by state and federal agencies.

INSURED REQUIRING HOSPITAL/MEDICAL CARE

Not too critical of charges because of "Oh well, our insurance is paying for it!" attitude.

NOT INSURED REQUIRING HOSPITAL/MEDICAL CARE — PAY OUT OF POCKET

Bad charges include "costs" not properly an obligation of patients: (1) Medical student and intern training; (2) "Research." These should be funded by state or federal government.

115

APPENDIX 2

WAR DEPARTMENT

FORT WAYNE ORDNANCE DEPOT

DETROIT, MICHIGAN

HARE/pr Ext. 1
10 December 1943

Mr. Rex Dye
Chairman, Control Staff
Fort Wayne
Detroit, Michigan

Dear Mr. Dye:

In looking back upon my tour of duty as Commanding Officer of Fort Wayne and in reflecting upon the quality of service of the many loyal and efficient civilian employees who have supported me, yours has been outstanding.

While you were employed originally as a Statistician, you have rapidly and steadily increased your value to this Depot until your position is tantamount to that of an efficiency and management engineer. As such, through your ability to analyze trends, and your foresight in anticipating bottlenecks, your recommendations for corrective action have not only been approved in a great majority of cases but have played an important part in the successful operation of this Depot.

I am mindful of the respect accorded your judgment and work by higher authority in the Army as is evidenced by the frequent calls we have had for your attendance at conferences.

Recently the Fort Wayne Post and Depot were called upon to nominate one civilian employee whom we considered best qualified for the Exceptional Civilian Service Award. You were the unanimous choice of the Committee and in that choice I concurred heartily.

I commend you for your initiative, your grasp of situations, your ability to act swiftly and for the wholehearted and enthusiastic support you have given me ever since you joined this Fort Wayne team.

Sincerely,

RAY M. HARE
Colonel, Ord. Dept.
Commanding

War Department

Army Service Forces

Commendation for Meritorious Civilian Service

To Whom It May Concern:

Rex Dye

has received official commendation and praise

for outstanding performance of duty

Citation:

In recognition of outstanding service at the Fort Wayne Ordnance Depot, Ordnance Department, Army Service Forces, in pioneering Control policy and procedure as applied to depot operations; in developing and refining Ordnance Depot report forms and content; in developing methods and procedures for management analysis of depot operations; in developing a Cost and Production Accounting System which brought about substantial increases in output per manhour; for carrying out these services on his own initiative and for using his own time in such service beyond his regular tour of duty.

Lieutenant General, Chief of Ordnance

Lieutenant General, Commanding

APPENDIX 4: HELPFUL ORGANIZATIONS

Common Cause
2030 M Street N.W.
Washington, D.C. 20036

Annual dues are $15.00 with a youth rate to anyone under 26 of $7.00 for first year membership.

Ralph Nader
Public Citizen, Inc.
P.O. Box 19404
Washington, D.C. 20036

APPENDIX 5

Regents, University of Michigan, list furnished by Allen M. Bennett, legislative analyst of the Republican office, House of Representatives at Lansing, Michigan. The "Memo to Regents" was sent to this list.

Brown, Paul W.
First Nat'l Bank Bldg.
Petoskey, Michigan 49770

Brown, Robert J.
no address given

Cudlip, William B.
800 First Nat'l Bldg.
Detroit, Michigan 48226

*Dunn, Gerald R.
15125 Farmington Rd.
Livonia, Michigan 48154

---

*Mr. Dunn unsuccessfully tried to get the veil of secrecy removed from salaries paid at University of Michigan and University Hospital. Only one other regent supported his proposal.

Huebner, Gertrude V.
no address given

Lindemer, Lawrence B.
900 Am. Bank & Trust Bldg.
Lansing, Michigan 48933

Nederlander, Robert E.
2555 Guardian Bldg.
Detroit, Michigan 48226

Waters, James L.
175 W. Apple at 1st
P.O. Box 27
Muskegon, Michigan 49443

Recommendations
for Further Reading

Sylvia A. Law, *Blue Cross: What Went Wrong?* (Yale University Press, 92 A Yale Station, New Haven, Connecticut 06520)

Prepared by the Health Law Project, University of Pennsylvania. A valuable study of the relation of Blue Cross to the present crisis in health care as a financing arm of American hospitals, accountable to neither the public nor its subscribers. An important book, well documented.

Ruth Winter, *How to Reduce Your Medical Bills* (Crown Publishers, Inc., 419 Park Avenue South, New York, N.Y. 10016)

The author is the wife of a medical doctor and she is a science editor of the *Newark Star Ledger*. She cites one case where a seven-hour stay in Dover General Hospital, Dover, N.J., ending in death for the patient resulted in a hospital bill of $2,124.55—over $300 an hour—and the hospital placed a lien for the full amount on the parents' home. She discusses hospital board trustees selling land to hospitals, bill-padding by hospitals, excessive pay to pathologists and radiologists. Well researched and highly informative.

Edward M. Kennedy, *In Critical Condition: The Crisis in America's Health Care* (Simon and Schuster, 630 Fifth Avenue, New York, N.Y. 10020)

This book is an indictment of the American health industry. Based on the senator's hearings as Chairman of the Senate Health Committee, the book cites case after case dealing with the tragedy of illness and the greed of health care suppliers. He deals with the exorbitant charges for hospital service, the evils of Blue Cross, monopolistic practices in the health market and the dollar motivation of hospitals. This book is shocking and cases cited are well documented.

C. Northcote Parkinson, *Law of Delay: Interviews and Outer-views* (Houghton, Mifflin Company, 2 Park Street, Boston, Massachusetts 02107)

An invaluable book for those who wish an insight into the manner in which politicians and bureaucrats operate. It sheds an interesting light on such political studies as the 500-page "study" by Michigan Governor Milliken's "Technical Work Group" on health care costs titled "Rising Medical Costs in Michigan: The Report of the Secretary's Commission on Medical Malpractice" and its 870 page (8½ × 11 page size in small type!) "appendix" by the Department of Health, Education and Welfare and "Hearings Before the Subcommittee on Antitrust and Monopoly," dealing with the high cost of hospitalization, of which Senator Philip A. Hart, Michigan, was chairman. Over the past four years millions of words of "studies," "reports" and generalized "recommendations" have been written and published at taxpayer expense by politicians and bureaucrats—but action has not been taken to correct the condition, in fact it is getting critically worse!

Parkinson's *Law of Delay* shows how and why this happens and is so interesting it's hard to put down after you have read a few pages.

William Proxmire, *Uncle Sam—The Last of the Big Time Spenders* (Simon and Schuster, 630 Fifth Avenue, New York, N.Y. 10020)

In chapter 6 and chapter 9 the senator tells how doctors are "making a killing" through Medicare and how the head of the Antibiotics Division of the FDA served the drug industry (and himself) for seven years while on the public payroll. He states that it is a truism that the great departments of government routinely act on behalf of the major economic interests under their jurisdiction rather than in the public interest. With such a condition at the national level what can be expected at the level of state and municipal governments?

This book is timely and devastating. It gives the reader a shocking picture of how his or her tax dollars are used by profligate politicians and who gets the money.

Index

"Action Line," *Detroit Free Press*, 35-36, 110

American Hospital Association, 71

American Medical Association, 81, 89, 107

American Medical Political Action Committee, 89

Ball, Robert M., 94-95

Beaumont General Hospital, Detroit, 36

Bed charges, 16

Bennett, Alan M., 61

Beverly Manor Convalescent Center, 28-30, 62

Blue Cross, 36, 42-43, 72, 108

Blue Cross Association, 71

Broomfield, William S. (M.C.), 78-80

Burn Center, University Hospital (Ann Arbor), 9

Campbell, Judge Ross W., 8, 18-19

Center magazine, 54

Children's Hospital (Detroit), 11

Committee on Ways and Means, House of Representatives, Washington, D.C., 86

Common Cause, 107, 110

Conflict of interest, 108

Connors, Edward M., 8, 31, 50, 57, 71, 105

Cost of hospitalization, 16-18, 39, 49, 58

Department of Health, Education and Welfare, U.S., 11, 49, 93-94

Department of Justice, U.S., Antitrust Division, 74

Department of Labor, U.S., 32

Detroit Chamber of Commerce, 74, 103

Detroit Free Press, 7-11, 13-14, 35-36, 38, 45-48, 110-11

Detroit Insurance Agency, 40

Doctor shortage, 52-53

Excessive bed time, 16-17

Excessive laboratory charges, 16

Flemming, Robben (President, Univ. of Mich.), 8

Food and Drug Administration, U.S., 10

Ford Motor Company, 37, 43

Frutig, Judith (*Detroit Free Press*), 47

Graff, Louis (University Hospital, Ann Arbor), 22-27

Grayson, C. Jackson, Jr. (Price Commission, U.S.), 96

Griffin, Senator, Robert P. (Mich.), 86-89

Griffiths, Representative Martha W. (Mich.), 76-78

Hall, Edward T., *The Silent Language,* 22

Hart, Senator Philip A. (Mich.), 50, 69-75

Heath, Mott B. (Ford Motor Co.), 101-2

122

Henry Ford Hospital, Detroit, 45
Holmes, Susan (*Detroit Free Press*), 45-46

Iacocca, Lee A. (Ford Motor Co.), 100-101
Insurance bureau, state of Mich., 41-42
Insurance principles, 40-42, 112

Kanby, Dr. Arnold H., 9
Katz, Dolores (*Detroit Free Press*), 38, 48
Kefauver Investigating Committee, 10
Kelley, Frank (Attorney General, Mich.), 66-69
Kennedy, Senator Edward M. (N.Y.), 37, 107
Kernodle, Dr. John F., 7, 81, 103
Ketchum, Dr. Jesse, 11, 106
Knowles, Dr. John F., 7, 71, 77-78, 103
Korszybski, Alfred, 25

Landers, Ann, 13
Law, Sylvia, 43
Lewis, Dr. W. J. (Chairman, American Medical Political Action Committee), 89
Lin, Paul T. K. ("Medicine in China," *Center* magazine), 54
Lobby funds, A.M.A., 107

McCann, Claude, 41
McDonald, Jack, 83-86
McKenna (Ford Motor Co.), 37, 100
Malpractice, 54, 105
Massachusetts Medical Society, 7
Materna, Michael (assistant attorney general, Mich.), 8
Medicaid fraud, 11
Medical Encyclopedia, Inc., 10

"Medicine in China" (Paul T. K. Lin, *Center magazine*), 54
Michigan Medicaid, 38
Michigan Medicare, 11
Michigan State University, 50, 102-3
Milliken, Governor William G., 56-60, 102
Monopoly in the health market, 38
Mt. Clemens General Hospital, 36

Nader, Ralph, 106, 110
Neeb, Louis P. (Price Commission, Washington, D.C.), 96-98
Noel, Governor Philip W. (R.I.), 81
Northville Record, 39, 52

Ogilvie, Governor Richard B. (Illinois), 9
Osteopaths, 53-54, 106
Overloading appointments, 12, 113

Padding bills, 37, 106
Pathologists' "take," 39, 71
Patterson, L. Brooks (prosecuting attorney, Oakland County, Mich.), 11
Payne, Dr. James D., 11
Petersburg General Hospital (Virginia), 10
Physical therapy, 17, 24
Price Commission, Executive Office of the President, 96
Providence Hospital (Detroit), 47
Proxmire, Senator William (Wisc.), 10
Purcell, Senator Carl D. (Mich.), 65-66

Roth, Russel B. (President, American Medical Association), 81

St. Joseph Hospital (Pontiac, Mich.), 47

Secrecy, 39, 50, 78, 111

Silent Language, The, Edward T. Hall, 22

Sinai Hospital (Detroit), 35, 37

Smart, Senator Clifford (Mich.), 60-63

Social Security Administration, 43, 91

Southern Illinois Hospital Corporation, 9

Sparrow Hospital (Lansing, Mich.), 35

Taylor, Dr. James B., 9

"Technical Work Group on Health Care Costs," 58

Tsutsumida, Cherry Y. (H.E.W.), 82

University Center, 9

University Hospital (Ann Arbor, Mich.), 8, 9, 13-34, 36, 42, 46-47, 56, 112

University of Michigan, 8, 13, 53

University of Pennsylvania, 43

Vienna, David P., 9

Violation of privacy, 17, 53

Virtue, Mrs. Maxine Boord (Assistant Attorney General, Mich.), 68

Vitu, Dr. Robert (President, Mich. Academy of Family Practice), 39, 52-53

Washtenaw News Review, 11, 31-32, 71

Wayne State University, 53

Weinberger, Casper M., 11

Welch, Dr. Henry (Food and Drug Administration), 10

Winter, Mrs. Ruth, 38, 106

Wolf, Fred B., 92-93

Wolfe, Dr. Sidney, 105

Ziem, Judge Frederick C., 11

Zollar, Senator Charles (Mich.), 63-64

Zugich, John J. (Associate Director, University Hospital, Ann Arbor, Mich.), 16, 18, 20-21